CHANGING AMERICA'S HEALTH CARE SYSTEM
Proposals for Legislative Action

SHELAH LEADER
and
MARILYN MOON,
Editors

With Contributions by
KAREN DAVIS
ALAIN ENTHOVEN
ROBERT EVANS
ROBERT KANE

An AARP Book published by
The Public Policy Institute
American Association of Retired Persons, Washington, D.C.
Scott, Foresman and Company, Glenview, Illinois

Library of Congress Cataloging-in-Publication Data

Changing America's health care system : proposals for legislative
    action / Shelah Leader and Marilyn Moon, editors ; with
    contributions by Karen Davis . . . [et al.].
        p.   cm.
    Includes bibliographies and index.
    1. Medical care—United States—Forecasting.   2. Medical care—
    Government policy—United States.   I. Leader, Shelah Gilbert.   II. Moon,
Marilyn.   III. Davis, Karen.
    RA395.A3C473 1989
    362.1'0973—dc19   88-17744
                                                                          CIP

1 2 3 4 5 6 RRC 93 92 91 90 89 88

ISBN 0-673-24895-X

AARP BOOKS provides interesting, timely, and practical information that enables
persons 50 and over to improve the quality of their lives in their health, housing,
finances, recreation, personal relationships, and work environment. These books
are copublished by AARP, the world's largest membership and service organization
for people 50 and over, and Scott, Foresman and Company, one of the nation's
foremost educational publishers. For further information, contact AARP Books,
1900 East Lake Avenue, Glenview, IL 60025.

CONTENTS

ACKNOWLEDGMENTS

Barbara Herzog, director of AARP's Health Care Campaign, provided the essential ingredients for this undertaking—enthusiasm, creative ideas, and funding. We would like to express our sincere appreciation for her unflagging support. The workshop and this book were a cooperative endeavor by AARP's Program and Field Services Division, headed by Anne Harvey, and the Division of Legislation, Research, and Public Policy under John Rother. We would like to thank them both for all their help. Finally, we would especially like to thank Barbara Goodwin and Kay Rose for cheerfully helping us see the project to fruition.

Shelah Leader
Marilyn Moon

FOREWORD

The issue of health care—its cost, its quality, and the lack of access to it—is again moving to center stage in America. The United States is the only industrialized nation other than South Africa without health insurance for all its citizens. An estimated 37 million Americans, including 11 million children, have no basic health coverage today. And almost all Americans lack adequate protection against the ravages of health care costs for long-term chronic conditions.

Although many claim that we have the best medical care in the world, that care is too often unavailable to those without insurance. Blocking moves toward more universal access to care are the runaway costs of the expensive system now in place. Inflation in health care costs has consistently outpaced inflation in the rest of the economy by two to three times in the last ten years. Currently the U.S. spends 11 percent of its GNP on health care, with most experts predicting continued sharp increases unless strong reforms are enacted.

Recent efforts to cut the rising cost of the Medicare program have, however, raised serious concerns about quality issues. New studies reveal a disturbing lack of agreement within the medical profession as to the proper treatment for certain conditions, and many doctors are said to be overtreating and subjecting patients to unnecessary surgery. Malpractice remains a serious concern in many parts of the country. Businesses have begun to cut back on coverage and experiment with a variety of new delivery organizations in efforts to control costs and protect quality.

In the wake of the national debate over catastrophic health coverage for older and disabled Americans, Congress seems prepared to recognize at last the failures due to our lack of a long-term care insurance and delivery system. Disabled and chronically ill Americans of all ages today must face tragic choices between needed care and other family needs. We have a system that forces most persons unfortunate enough to have illnesses such as Alzheimer's disease to give up a lifetime of hard won economic security and see themselves and their families forced into welfare.

Recent polls indicate that Americans of all ages are growing impatient with inaction and are looking to their elected leaders to address the whole range of health care concerns. The growing recognition that the status quo is not working for many American families is sparking a renewed interest in major reform.

What's needed now is a credible and practical approach to solving these problems. Many suggest that we look north, to Canada, to learn from a country that seems to have solved many of these issues. Others suggest that greater reliance on tightly controlled means of competition and greater consumer choice within the health insurance system would produce economies and more sensible decisions at the local level. Still others rely on the expansion of the present division of responsibility between the private and public sectors, with mandated health coverage for those working and expanded public sector programs for those not working.

We stand at a crossroads on these policy directions. We cannot afford to wait much longer to address the needs, or the problems will grow even more difficult. The debate must be joined, it must be comprehensive, and it must make sense to the American people. For that reason I commend the American Association of Retired Persons for bringing together outstanding thinkers in this book to challenge themselves and each other to articulate a national health reform agenda. I hope this volume will help forge a new political consensus on how to make health care the universal right most Americans want—not the day after tomorrow, but tomorrow.

Dr. Arthur Flemming
Former Secretary, U.S. Department of
Health, Education, and Welfare
Co-chair, Save Our Security: Coalition to
Protect Social Security

INTRODUCTION

This book culminates a project first conceived in the spring of 1986 when several of us on the AARP staff confessed to each other our yearning to reflect quietly on the type of health care system we as a nation should be creating. If only, we agreed, we shared a common vision of a future society, we'd be better able to shape policy rather than simply react to short-term political demands and crises. We worried that the cumulative effect of multiple marginal changes we supported would be an inadequate whole.

Upon further thought, we agreed that the opportunity to brainstorm with a few respected experts would be an excellent way to clarify our long-term goals and options.

Ultimately, the following process was devised. Four health policy experts were invited to write essays on their own vision of a better health care delivery system. Essentially, they were asked to devise a blueprint for AARP's health-related action over the next ten years.

In selecting the experts, we sought out respected scholars who are each well known as advocates of a particular plan or approach to reforming the U.S. health care system. We tried to choose advocates of a broad variety of approaches within a range that is basically compatible with AARP's own policies and values. Therefore, we did not choose an advocate of a totally privatized delivery system because dismantling Medicare would be quite unacceptable to AARP members.

Accordingly, Professors Karen Davis of Johns Hopkins, Alain Enthoven of Stanford, Robert Evans of the University of British Columbia, and Robert Kane of the University of Minnesota were invited to propose a way to restructure our health care system for the benefit of all persons, with particular emphasis on older Americans.

Each was asked to propose a plan and specify the basic philosophy or value system behind that plan. Specifics were to include the financing method; the quality-control mechanisms; the roles of consumers, providers, and the government; the expected cost controls; the plan's comprehensiveness; the organization of care; the provision of long-term care; and the roles of Medicare and Medicaid.

These proposals were then circulated among the experts, the AARP volunteer leaders, and the AARP staff with responsibility for health care policy and programs.

Since we particularly wanted to obtain a systematic critique of each expert's proposal, we built into the process a requirement that each agree to be criticized—in public—by a peer. Traditionally, busy and well-known experts pass each other on the conference and congressional talk circuit. They may take pot shots at each other's views on a public platform, but they rarely participate in a forum where their ideas are subjected to rigorous and sustained analysis according to criteria established by consumers.

Therefore, we created the basis for debate by asking Evans to criticize Davis, Davis to criticize Kane, Enthoven to critique Evans, and Kane to critique Enthoven. We tried to assign responsibility for the critic's role to the strongest likely opponent of each proposal.

The critiques had to specifically address the following points:

- the merits of the proposal,
- its feasibility,
- likely unintended or unanticipated consequences,
- key erroneous assumptions,
- unaddressed issues,
- cost control and financing, and
- quality of care and access to services.

Again, the written critiques were circulated prior to the formal workshop held on December 7-9, 1986.

The experts agreed to participate in this workshop where they could defend their views against the criticism of their plan as well as against the probing questions of invited AARP volunteers and staff. The experts were told that they could revise their proposals after the discussions, if they were moved to do so. And they knew that their written work and the discussion proceedings would be published.

We all met as planned for intense talks that lasted nearly two days and nights. The formal sessions were recorded by a court reporter, and the quotes in Chapter 8 are derived from the meeting transcripts. But the discussion proved so fascinating that it spilled beyond the planned sessions and continued during meals, breaks, and into the night. Unfortunately, these unscheduled exchanges are not recorded, but they accelerated the pace of the formal talks. At other times, we were unable to make progress on certain agenda items because the participants could not agree or simply didn't know how to solve particular conceptual or financial problems.

In other words, the transcripts do not reveal an entirely orderly and logical discussion. But they do show areas of consensus and some insight into the difficulties of planning for a better society. In compiling chapter 8, we have drawn from the official record to share the flavor and content of this fascinating undertaking.

Chapter 9 was written by Robert Evans after the meeting, and he neatly summarizes the drawbacks in the incremental changes advocated by Davis, Kane, and Enthoven. As our foreign participant-observer, Evans provides a Canadian perspective on our own system and reminds us that we have much to learn from other countries in meeting the health care needs of society.

In addition to the four health policy experts already named, the following six volunteer leaders were present:

Gwendolyn Bedford: Member, AARP's Board of Directors; officer of the Arizona Council for Senior Citizens; member of the Board of Governors of the Central Arizona Health Systems Agency; past chair of the Phoenix Public Housing Advisory Board; and member of the Mayor's Aging Services Commission.

Louise Crooks: President-elect of AARP; a delegate to the 1985 U.N. Conference on Women in Nairobi, Kenya; and former president of the Indiana Retired Teachers Association. She taught public school for thirty-one years.

George Engelter: Member, AARP's Board of Directors; chair of AARP's Voter Education Fund; former manager of newspaper-owned radio stations; and former director of the North Dakota Motor Carrier's Association.

Clarice Jones: Past chair of AARP's Board of Directors; delegate to the 1950 and 1960 White House Conference on Children and Youth; and past president of the Michigan Association of Child Guidance Clinics.

Eugene Lehrmann: Member, AARP's Board of Directors; former president of Wisconsin Retired Teachers Association; legislative chair of the Wisconsin Coalition of Aging Groups; member of the advisory council to Wisconsin's Hospital Rate Setting Commission; and former president of the American Vocational Association.

C. Kermit Phelps, Ph.D.: Chair of AARP's Board of Directors; former chief clinical psychologist at the Veterans Administration Hospital in Kansas City; and former officer of the Missouri Psychological Association, the National Conference of Christians and Jews, and his county Civil Rights Commission.

AARP staff attending were Jack Christy, Frank Forbes, Robert Harootyan, Anne Harvey, Barbara Herzog, Shelah Leader, Charlotte Mahoney, Cheryl Matheis, Greg Merrill, Marilyn Moon, Bette Mullen, Tom Nelson, Barbara Quaintance, John Rother, Sana Shtasel, Patricia Smith, Jane Tilly, and Theresa Varner. All of these staff members work on health research, policy, and programs for the Association.

Prior commitments prevented AARP's then president, John Denning, and then executive director, Cyril F. Brickfield, from attending the meeting.

To our knowledge, this project represents a unique effort by a major membership organization of consumers (28 million members and growing) to identify a long-term policy goal and appropriate strategy.

By sharing this process with you, we hope to provoke a broader national debate on the flaws of our current health care system and the direction of needed change.

CONTRIBUTORS

Karen Davis, Ph.D., is chair of the Department of Health Policy and Management, Johns Hopkins University School of Hygiene and Public Health. She was formerly a senior fellow at the Brookings Institute and then served as deputy assistant secretary for planning and evaluation for health policy, Department of Health, Education, and Welfare, and as Administrator of the Health Resources Administration for the Public Health Service.

Alain Enthoven, Ph.D., is Marriner S. Eccles Professor, Graduate School of Business at Stanford University. He has worked for the RAND Corporation; was assistant secretary for systems analysis in the Department of Defense; and was an officer in Litton Industries.

Robert Evans, Ph.D., is professor of economics at the University of British Columbia, Canada. He has served as advisor to the provincial government of Ontario and as consultant to the Ministry of Health in Manitoba. He is also a member of the advisory committee of the National Health Research and Development program in Ottawa. He has written widely on the Canadian health care system.

Robert Kane, M.D., is the dean at the School of Public Health, University of Minnesota. He was formerly a senior researcher at the RAND Corporation and a professor at the UCLA Schools of Medicine and Public Health. He serves as a consultant to a number of national and international agencies including the National Institute on Aging, the National Center for Health Services Research, the Institute of Medicine, and the World Health Organization.

Shelah Leader, Ph.D., is a health policy analyst with AARP's Public Policy Institute. She was a senior research analyst in the U.S. Department of Health and Human Services and director of research and education for the National Consumers League.

Marilyn Moon, Ph.D., is director of AARP's Public Policy Institute. She was formerly a senior research associate at the Urban Institute and a senior research analyst at the Congressional Budget Office. She has also taught economics at the University of Wisconsin–Milwaukee.

1

THE U.S. HEALTH CARE SYSTEM OF THE FUTURE: A LONG-RANGE POLICY PROPOSAL

Karen Davis

In recent years health policy in the United States has been shaped through the annual federal budget process. Large budget deficits and the tactic of including all major legislative changes in Medicare and Medicaid in an omnibus reconciliation bill have changed the nature of health policy deliberations. The short time frame during which the president's budget is considered and a reconciliation bill is passed by the Congress puts an emphasis on incremental and short-term health policy changes. Measures are passed that yield either real or illusionary immediate savings, including provisions that shift outlays from one budgetary period to another or from the federal government to state governments or the private sector. Annual changes in health programs are not developed in the context of a long-range health policy framework. In addition, health policy is no longer primarily driven by goals for health, but rather by federal budgetary goals. Such a process leads to neither good health policy nor good budgetary policy.

Health policy is no longer primarily driven by goals for health, but rather by federal budgetary goals. Such a process leads to neither good health policy nor good budgetary policy.

The United States needs a policy debate over the nature of the health care system we wish to have in the future. Once the parties agree on this longer-term policy framework, they can take steps on an annual basis that will be consistent with this longer-term plan. To advance such a debate, this paper sets forth one vision of a long-range plan for health policy in the United States. This plan could be achieved over time with a series of legislative and budgetary measures enacted on an annual basis; desired elements of the overall plan could be phased in over time as budgetary resources permit and as experience with each step is gained.

The plan advanced here is incremental in nature. The primary advantage of an incremental approach is its adaptability to the federal budget process, which constantly weighs competing budget priorities. New initiatives are feasible in a tight budget framework, but only if they are relatively modest in scope. Current programs are familiar to legislators, fall within clearly defined jurisdictional boundaries, and have advocates among members of authorizing committees. Brand new programs that are sweeping in nature are too filled with uncertainty to be acted upon on a tight legislative calendar.

There is, of course, a downside to this incremental strategy. More attractive elements of a long-term package may be enacted first, leaving no momentum for further change. To have administrative systems maintaining multiple programs may be more complex than designing a new system from scratch. Tight cost-control measures may also be more difficult to coordinate among multiple programs, which can be played off against each other by providers.

If political and economic conditions permit a major large-scale reform, the plan proposed here could be enacted in a single step or in several large steps. It is, in that sense, adaptable to either strategy.

GOALS FOR THE U.S. HEALTH CARE SYSTEM

The United States was founded for the purpose of assuring life, liberty, and the pursuit of happiness for all. We seek to create a humane society that values human life and that assures the right of all to live with dignity. This philosophy has especially important implications for the health sector, which is so essential to achieving this lofty purpose.

Achievement of multiple goals often requires compromise. Goals may be in conflict. Most typically the desire to control costs runs counter to goals to improve access or quality of care. Acceptability and freedom to choose among alternatives may also be in conflict with goals of limiting costs. More basically, assuring a decent life for all, for example, may impinge on individual liberty, as resources are transferred within the society to ensure a minimum standard of living for all. In a world of constrained resources, trade-offs must be made among multiple goals, some of which are in conflict. However, as a basis for evaluating alternative policy directions for the future, it is helpful to be explicit about those goals that most Americans want to see their health sector achieve. As a starting point, the following goals are set forth.

Goal 1

Reduce preventable mortality and morbidity. The World Health Organization (WHO) has urged the adoption of "Health for All by the Year 2000" as a major goal of all countries. This goal calls for the maximum attainable health and social well-being of the population, presumably within the constraint of a reasonable level of economic resources devoted to the health sector. The United States, along with other nations around the world, has committed itself to achieving major improvement in the health of the population by the end of the century. The U.S. commitment was embodied in the report of the Surgeon General under the Carter administration, entitled *Healthy People*, and was renewed in presentations before the World Health Assembly by the Surgeon General under the Reagan administration. In response to the WHO initiative, the United States has established goals on reducing preventable mortality and morbidity by establishing a set of health objectives to be achieved through improvements in lifestyles, reduction in occupational and environmental hazards, and accessibility of preventive health care services to the entire population. Fiscal support of this initiative, however, has been sharply curtailed under the Reagan administration.

Goal 2

Quality of Life: Enhance the quality of life at the end of the lifespan by maintaining functioning capacity as long as possible, ensuring relief of avoidable pain and discomfort, and allowing control over choices affecting the manner of living and dying. As the population of the United States is aging, more attention is being given by ethicists to the quality of life at the end of the lifespan. Some health conditions are terminal in nature and require primarily hospice care to relieve pain and assist the individual and his or her family in making the most of the time remaining. Other chronic conditions such as Alzheimer's disease lead to a slow deterioration in mental or physical functioning. For those with such conditions the primary goal should be to maintain functioning capacity as long as possible, to provide support for the patient and family, and to guarantee patients and families control over major decisions affecting the nature of care (e.g., whether or not to be in a nursing home or to receive high-technology care).

Goal 3

Access: Assure that no one is denied health care because of an inability to pay. One of the most important social goals is to assure adequate access to health care services for the entire population. This is particularly important for the most vulnerable members of society. The poor, for example, are unable to afford costly health care without assistance. Similarly, individuals at high risk—such as AIDS victims—may be excluded from insurance coverage without special provisions. Patients with complex problems—for example, those requiring total parenteral nutrition—may be refused treatment by hospitals paid a fixed rate for all patients with a given diagnosis. An equitable health care system would assure that no one is turned away from care because of high risk or inability to pay.

Goal 4

Equitable Financing: Assure that the financial burden of health care expenses is equitably distributed. No one should suffer financial hardship by being required to pay health bills that are high in relation to family income. Catastrophic illness can pose a hardship for nearly everyone; even minor illnesses or accidents can result in serious financial hardship to the uninsured poor.

Goal 5

Costs: Promote efficiency and effectiveness in the provision of health care services. Despite the high expectations that Americans have for their health sector, they are also concerned with high outlays for health care. They would like to see improvements in productivity and efficiency in the health sector by eliminating waste or unnecessary services, containing excess profits, and in general, assuring that health benefits are received in proportion to money spent on health care.

Goal 6

Quality of Care and Technological Progress: Preserve and enhance the quality of health care. Americans have come to expect and demand high-quality health care. They expect physicians to recommend a course of diagnosis and treatment that is in their best interest and that will best assure their well-being. They expect hospitals and other health facilities to be adequately equipped and staffed with qualified, trained personnel and to be committed to the delivery of appropriate care. They expect their physicians to be dedicated, well trained, and highly qualified. If a new technology—such as heart or liver transplants—works, they expect to obtain it when needed.

Americans expect continual progress in all sectors of society. Maintenance of quality of care is not sufficient. Continued advancement of knowledge, breakthroughs in biomedical research, and technological progress are widely desired.

Goal 7

Freedom to Choose: Maintain the right to make choices individually or collectively through a democratic political process. Individual rights are an integral part of the American culture. Americans expect to be informed about choices affecting their lives and well-being and to have the ultimate say in those decisions. They feel strongly about the right to choose their own physician or health delivery system and to be able to vote with their feet if they are dissatisfied with the care or advice they are receiving.

The American political system is a democracy. Just as individuals want the right to make individual choices, they expect the right to make some decisions on a collective basis through a democratic political process. Choices made individually through the marketplace are not inherently more sacrosanct than choices made collectively through the political process.

Clearly, expecting to achieve all seven of these social goals completely is unrealistic. Policy options that create incentives for efficiency and productivity may lead health care providers to cut corners and lead to some deterioration in the quality of care. As a society, if informed of these trade-offs, we may well choose in some instances to obtain lower costs even if it entails more inconvenience, or to pay more to assure that everyone has access to care.

EVALUATING POLICY OPTIONS

Any policy option should be evaluated in terms of whether it does or does not contribute to the social goals set forth above. While different individuals may weigh the importance of these goals differently, a thorough analysis of policy options should indicate the impact the option would have on access, equity, health, quality of life, quality of care, progress, and free choice as well as the implications for the cost of care and its distribution among alternative sources of financing.

Costs

Any policy proposal should be evaluated with a clear understanding of its costs—including additional real economic resources that must be diverted to the health sector and the budgetary cost to different levels of government. Estimates should also be available on costs shifted from the public sector to the private sector, or the reverse, and on any change in cost to different individuals. Estimates of economic and budgetary costs should be available both for the point of implementation and over time.

Acceptability

Patients expect health care cost-containment initiatives to result in lower out-of-pocket expenses for health care; yet, some policy approaches such as increased cost sharing in employer health plans take the opposite tack. If policy options are to be viable in the long term, they need to correspond with patient expectations. The initiative needs to be simple enough to be easily understood. Similarly, physicians and other health care providers need to find the policy option acceptable to avoid mass opposition or boycotting of the program.

The central element of my long-range policy proposal is universal health insurance coverage achieved through expansions in coverage under existing public and private health insurance plans.

Administrative Feasibility

Any policy option should be relatively easy to administer. This puts a premium on incremental changes that build on current systems of financing. Simplicity of the program is to be desired—both for ease of understanding and for administrative purposes.

Political Feasibility

Finally, policy options need to be able to muster political support from major interest groups—labor, business, insurance, physicians, hospitals, and consumer groups such as senior citizens' organizations and advocacy groups. Political support from all geographical regions is important, as is support from state and local government officials. While a consensus of all parties is extraordinarily difficult to obtain, accommodation to major concerns can help mitigate opposition.

The long-range policy proposal presented here has the following characteristics:

- It is designed to make major gains in the achievement of the goals set forth above.
- It is incremental in nature, but it presents a vision of the ultimate desired system. It attempts to improve the existing system of health care financing and organization rather than replace it.
- It assumes that implementation of the long-range policy proposal will be achieved in phases over time rather than through a single legislative measure.

The criteria of administrative and political feasibility, in particular, rules out the wholesale adoption of health financing systems from other countries. This means that the proposal accepts a mixed public–private system of financing health services. I assume that health care services in the United States will continue to be provided predominantly by private nonprofit or for-profit organizations and that physicians will continue to have the option of selecting from a mix of fee-for-service and prepaid modes of practice.

My proposal primarily emphasizes reform of health care financing, including health insurance coverage for acute and long-term care services and reform of methods of paying physicians, hospitals, and other health care providers. It also includes incentives to reform the organization and delivery of health care services to promote efficiency and quality of care. I believe it could be achieved over the next ten years.

ACUTE HEALTH CARE INSURANCE COVERAGE

The central element of my long-range policy proposal is universal health insurance coverage achieved through expansions in coverage under existing public and private health insurance plans. Employer-provided health plans for those in the workforce and their dependents are expanded, the elderly and disabled are covered under Medicare, and Medicaid is expanded to cover all others.

Employer Mandate

Coverage of all full-time workers and their dependents under employer health plans would be mandatory, and minimum benefit standards would be prescribed. Standards would apply to all firms, whether firms elected to self-insure or to purchase coverage through health insurers. Specifically, employers' plans would have to meet the following criteria.

Eligibility

Employers with twenty or more full-time employees would be required to cover all these employees, their spouses, and dependents. Full-time is defined as persons who have worked twenty-five hours per week for ten consecutive weeks. No worker or dependent could be denied coverage, nor could preexisting conditions be excluded from coverage.

Extension of Coverage

Coverage would begin after the tenth week of employment and must continue at least ninety days after termination of employment or after the death of a worker or divorce of a worker and spouse. During this period, the employer would continue to share in the premium cost. Employees and their dependents would have to be given the right to buy comparable individual-plan coverage at group rates after this period for as long as they choose to pay the full group-premium cost plus 2 percent administrative fee.

Benefits

The minimum benefit package must include inpatient hospital services; physician and other ambulatory services without arbitrary limits; preventive care including complete prenatal, delivery, and infant care without cost sharing; home health care (up to 100 visits per year); and limited mental health care. Employers could provide a broader benefit package but not less than the minimum.

Catastrophic Coverage

Proposed employer plans may include patient deductibles and coinsurance (with the exception of maternal and infant care), but cost sharing for a family may not exceed $2,500 annually, or $1,250 for an individual.

Annual deductibles may not exceed $500, and coinsurance rates may not exceed 25 percent.

Choice of HMO and PPO

All qualified employer plans must give employees and their dependents a choice of enrollment in any federally qualified Health Maintenance Organization (HMO) or a federally qualified Preferred Provider Organization (PPO) when those are available in the community and elect to be offered.

Financing

Employers would be required to pay at least 75 percent of premium costs for the mandated plan. Higher employer premium shares could, of course, be agreed to. Today, more than 85 percent of workers with employer-financed insurance are covered in plans where the employer pays at least 75 percent of the premium. Any employer whose premium contribution for a minimum plan exceeds 5 percent of payroll would be eligible for a tax credit to cover the excess cost. This would avoid an adverse economic impact on firms with low-wage workers.

Administration

Employer plans would be federally qualified and subject to state insurance regulatory provisions. Penalties would be assessed for mis-representation or nonconformance with federal standards.

Reinsurance

Employer plans, HMOs, and PPOs would be eligible to buy reinsurance protection against the costs of truly extraordinary illness (over $25,000 per covered person), thus providing protection for self-insured businesses.

Small Firms

Small firms would be given incentives to establish multiemployer trusts to offer group coverage. Those employees and dependents not covered by employer plans would be eligible for Medicaid by paying an actuarially fair premium.

Medicare

The Medicare program would be expanded to cover all persons aged sixty-five and over and all disabled individuals. For those elderly and disabled covered under employer plans, the employer plan would provide primary coverage with secondary coverage under Medicare. The Hospital Insurance (HI) part of Medicare and the Supplementary Medical Insurance (SMI) part would be merged administratively and financially. Specific provisions include the following:

Eligibility

The new Medicare program would cover everyone sixty-five or older (not just those covered by Social Security) and the permanently and totally disabled (those receiving any disability insurance payments). The current two-year waiting period for the disabled would be eliminated. The work history requirements that govern eligibility for Social Security benefits would not apply for Medicare. All beneficiaries would be automatically covered for the full range of Medicare benefits, not just HI benefits as at present.

Benefits

All the current Medicare benefits would continue in the new plan, but the limits on covered hospital days would be removed. Short-stay skilled nursing home benefits would be retained to provide posthospital care. Home health benefits and other nursing home care would be provided under a new long-term care benefit (see below). Deductible and coinsurance provisions for hospital and physician services would be continued. A new ceiling on out-of-pocket expenses for covered benefits would be incorporated, set initially at $1,250 per beneficiary and indexed over time with the growth in program expenditures. Expenses counting toward the maximum would include all out-of-pocket payments for hospital, physician, and other Medicare benefits. Once a beneficiary had paid $1,250 in a given year for these benefits, Medicare would cover all additional expenses.

Financing

The HI and SMI Medicare trust funds would be merged. The current HI payroll tax would be retained as a source of revenue for the new fund and would continue at its current legislated rate. General revenues currently projected to support SMI would be added to the fund, and the current SMI premium would be replaced with an income-related premium. This new Medicare premium would be set at 2.5 percent of taxable income of the enrollees and would be administered through the personal income tax system. The definition of income would be broadened to be consistent with Social Security provisions for taxing the Social Security benefits of higher-income elderly.

The new premium would be capped at $1,000 annually so that no beneficiary would be required to pay a premium exceeding 50 percent of the actuarial value of Medicare. A minimum annual premium of $100 would ensure that all elderly Americans made some contribution; this minimum premium would be deducted from Social Security checks of all elderly and disabled. Both the minimum and maximum premium rates would be indexed over time with increases in program expenditures. Additional revenues for the new Medicare Trust Fund would come from doubling the current tax on cigarettes. These funds would be earmarked for Medicare and added to the trust fund.

Medi-Help

The federal government would make available under the Medicare program its own Medi-Gap supplemental policy, called Medi-Help. Medi-Help would provide complete coverage of the cost-sharing provisions in the basic Medicare coverage as well as prescription drug coverage over a $100 deductible. The prescription drug benefit would encourage use of generic drugs and include incentives for efficiency. This coverage would be provided on an optional basis to all Medicare beneficiaries for a premium set to cover the actuarial value of the supplementary benefit package plus administrative costs.

Medicaid

The Medicaid program would be expanded to provide acute health care benefits to the entire population falling outside employer-mandated coverage and Medicare coverage. It would provide complete coverage to the poor and premium-financed coverage to others. Medicaid would be a secondary payer for individuals covered under employer plans or Medicare.

Eligibility

All individuals with incomes below the federal poverty level would be automatically covered under Medicaid. Coverage would not be subject to an assets test. Categorical restrictions would be removed so that single individuals and childless couples would be covered. In exchange for a premium set on a sliding scale with income, Medicaid acute care benefits would be available to those not eligible for coverage under employer plans. The premium would not exceed the actuarial value of the Medicaid benefit package, plus administrative costs.

Benefits

The Medicaid program would cover the current mandatory benefits plus prescription drugs without arbitrary limits on amount, duration, or scope of benefits. Unnecessary use of services would be discouraged through utilization review and prior authorization provisions. For individuals purchasing coverage with a sliding-scale premium, modest cost sharing provisions would be included.

Medicare Supplementation

For those Medicaid beneficiaries also covered by Medicare, Medicaid would pay the Medicare premium, pick up Medicare's cost-sharing requirements, and cover prescription drugs. Long-term care benefits currently provided through Medicaid would continue to be available (see below). These benefits would be covered without any charge to individuals with incomes below the poverty level. Medicare beneficiaries with incomes between the poverty level and twice the poverty level could purchase Medicaid supplemental coverage for a sliding-scale premium rather than purchasing Medi-Help, for which they would be expected to pay the full actuarially determined premium.

Financing and Administration

The net new costs of expanded Medicaid coverage would be met through federal general revenues. States, however, would continue to contribute to the cost of acute and long-term Medicaid coverage but would not incur any additional costs in the aggregate. This would require adjusting the existing matching rate to a lower level across all states. However, an individual state might face higher costs from expanded coverage. Administration of coverage for new beneficiaries would be handled through state Medicaid administrative procedures.

LONG-TERM CARE COVERAGE

A new long-term care benefit would be added to the Medicare program. This would include an improved home health benefit and a new nursing home benefit. This portion of Medicare would be financed with an income-related premium. Ten percent of all funds in the long-term care trust fund would be dedicated to direct grant programs for respite and other support services, Alzheimer's assessment centers, and other long-term care services. Medicaid would be retained as a residual program to cover cost sharing for poor long-term care beneficiaries on Medicare. Medicaid would also cover disabled individuals qualified to receive Supplemental Security Income cash assistance who may not meet the more stringent requirements of the disability insurance program and other poor not covered by Medicare.

Eligibility

All individuals eligible for Medicare would automatically be covered by the long-term care benefit. This includes all persons aged sixty-five and over and the permanently and totally disabled receiving disability insurance payments.

Benefits

Current Medicare restrictions that limit home health coverage to the homebound in unstable health conditions who require the intermittent services of a registered nurse or a physical therapist would be relaxed. Physician approval would continue to be required. However, home health benefits would be subject to a 10 percent coinsurance charge.

Nursing home care would be covered by Medicare after two years of residence. The cost of the first two years would be paid either directly by patients or by their private insurance plans. After the first two years, patients would be required to contribute 10 percent of the cost of care up to an annual ceiling of $3,000.

Financing

The Medicare long-term care benefit would be financed by a mandatory income-related premium set to cover the actuarial cost of coverage. This is estimated to be about 2 percent of income, with a minimum premium of $200 and a maximum premium of $1,000. Private insurance companies would be encouraged to market plans to cover the cost of the first two years, subject to federal standards.

Direct Grants

Ten percent of the long term care premium funds would be dedicated to providing grants to increase the availability of services, provide information to families, assure the quality of care, and provide some respite and other support services. This would include the establishment of regional Alzheimer's centers to provide state-of-the-art diagnosis and care plans for Alzheimer's patients, Alzheimer's information hotlines and support groups, and support to nonprofit organizations providing respite services to families of Alzheimer's patients and others maintained at home requiring extensive home help assistance. Funds could also be used to develop day hospital or adult day care programs and improvements in the quality of home health and nursing home care.

Medicaid

Medicaid would continue to provide long-term care benefits. This would include coverage of all elderly and disabled individuals with incomes below the federal poverty level. Benefits would include complete nursing home care and home and community-based services. Federal matching rates would continue at the current rate of these services. Improved Medicare long-term care benefits would result in savings to states that would offset the increased cost of the Medicaid acute-care benefit and eligibility expansions.

SYSTEM REFORM

Medicare, Medicaid, and employer plans would be required to offer the choice of a federally qualified HMO if locally available. Federally qualified HMOs would be closely monitored to assure quality of care and fiscal soundness. A federal qualification process would be developed for preferred provider organizations to assure quality of care and fiscal soundness. Greater emphasis would be given to prevention and primary care programs through direct grant support.

Health Maintenance Organizations

Multiple HMO options would be offered wherever possible. No more than half the beneficiaries in any given HMO could be Medicare and Medicaid beneficiaries. HMOs would be required to offer a minimum-benefits package, as under current HMO law. They would be required to have open enrollment periods annually and enroll all applicants without regard to health risk or preexisting conditions. Medicare, Medicaid, and employer health plans would be required to provide clear, accurate, objective, and comprehensive information on options available to beneficiaries. Beneficiaries could not be charged a premium that depends upon their particular health risk or health status.

Prevention and Primary Care

The current health system is skewed toward specialized care and institutional care. Direct grant programs for prevention and primary care services would be expanded. Community health centers and migrant health centers would be expanded to meet the needs of disadvantaged population groups in medically underserved areas. Federal funds would be increased for prevention programs including immunizations and family planning services. Programs to encourage healthier lifestyles and to reduce injuries and exposure to harmful substances in the workplace, the environment, the community, and the home would be expanded.

PROVIDER PAYMENT REFORM

Major reforms in current methods of paying hospitals, physicians, and health maintenance organizations would be implemented. Payment under Medicaid and federally qualified preferred provider organizations would be tied to the Medicare provider payment methods.

Hospitals

The Diagnosis Related Group (DRG) prospective payment system for hospitals under Medicare would be retained and improved. Major modifications in the current system would include

- incorporating an additional percentage allowance in the DRG payment rate to cover the cost of capital;
- replacing the current direct medical education allowance with a per resident allowance varying with specialty;
- adjusting the DRG payment rate for inner city location, nonlabor costs, and hospitals that treat a disproportionate share of low-income patients;
- adjusting the DRG payment rate for teaching hospitals to take into account the complexity of cases treated;
- and setting the annual increase in the DRG payment rates for a three-year period through legislative action determined in a budgetary process that balances budgetary and health goals.

States would be encouraged to institute or maintain their own all-payer hospital prospective payment systems, generating at least the same level of budgetary savings as the DRG prospective payment system and assuring equity among payers.

Physicians

Physicians would be paid according to a fee schedule under Medicare. Relative values of the fee schedule would be based on the time required to provide a particular service with adjustment for skill or training required to provide the service. The level of the fee schedule would be set to be revenue-neutral, i.e., it would generate neither budgetary savings nor costs. Annual increases in the fee schedule would be pegged to increases in the Consumer Price Index. The fee schedule would be phased in by holding fees constant for those who otherwise would face a reduction in Medicare payment rates. All physicians would be required to accept assignment, i.e., they would not be permitted to charge patients fees in excess of the allowable fee.

HMOs

HMOs would be paid a capitated rate set on the basis of an actuarially fair premium. This would take into account the expected health utilization of the population enrolled, with appropriate adjustment for the health status of the enrolled population.

PPOs

To qualify as a federally qualified PPO, physicians, hospitals, and other health care providers could not charge a rate in excess of that provided under Medicare. In the case of hospitals, DRG prospective rates for nonelderly patients would be established. No hospital participating in the PPO could charge in excess of these rates. In the case of physicians, the Medicare allowable fee would be a maximum fee for any procedure.

Medicaid

Medicaid would follow Medicare payment rates for hospitals, physicians, and HMOs. The relative DRG prospective payment rates and levels could be adjusted to reflect the resource cost of caring for the nonelderly Medicaid population.

SUMMARY

My proposal would contribute to improved health of the population by removing financial barriers to medical care and increasing funding for prevention and primary care. Maternity and infant-care services would be covered without cost sharing for those covered by both employer plans and Medicaid. Improved access to acute care for the uninsured would improve health and give children a better chance at productive lives.

Improved long-term care benefits would provide greater choices for frail elderly and disabled persons. Respite services and specific services for patients with Alzheimer's disease or other burdensome chronic conditions would be provided.

Universal access to health care services would be guaranteed through coverage of the entire population under employer health plans, Medicare, or Medicaid. Coverage under both employer plans and Medicare would be expanded, leaving Medicaid as a safety net to cover any others and financed through federal general revenues and a sliding-scale premium. Employer plans, HMOs, and PPOs would not be permitted to exclude individuals with high risk or to charge such individuals higher premiums.

The proposal would lead to a more equitable distribution of the financial burden of health care expenses. Maximum out-of-pocket ceilings on health care expenses would be instituted in all plans. Limits on covered hospital days under Medicare would be removed. All persons with incomes below the federal poverty level would be eligible for complete coverage without cost sharing through the Medicaid program. New long-term care benefits under Medicare would eliminate the enormous financial hardship now faced by those in nursing homes and ease the problem of becoming impoverished before one can obtain benefits, as under means-tested Medicaid.

Incentives to control costs and improve efficiency would be accomplished through numerous provider payment and system reform provisions. All individuals would have a choice of enrollment in federally qualified HMOs. Prospective payment of hospital and physician services would be extended through PPOs and new provisions in Medicare and Medicaid.

Quality standards would be developed and monitored through Medicare, Medicaid, HMOs, and PPOs. Provider payment rates would be set to ensure continued room for technological progress and development. Quality standards for nursing homes would be improved with better federal financial control.

Individuals would be given information and choices among alternative health plans. Public financing would be targeted on the poor and those falling outside employer plans.

Precise cost estimates of the long-range proposal are not now available. The major new governmental outlays to be financed through taxes would be for expanded coverage of the poor under Medicaid. This would entail substantial new outlays. Long-term care benefits and acute-care benefit improvements in Medicare would be financed through income-related premiums paid by beneficiaries.

The long-range policy proposal builds on current programs and continues current administrative mechanisms. For example, state agencies would continue to have responsibility for enrolling the poor in Medicaid. Policy regarding provider payment would be established by intermediaries under Medicare. Some new administrative mechanisms would need to be established, however, to monitor quality of care and fiscal soundness of a greater variety of health plans. More individuals would become eligible under Medicaid, and many smaller employers would be required to provide health insurance to workers and dependents for the first time. Income-related premiums for Medicare beneficiaries would be assessed through the personal income tax system and would require new administrative procedures.

The long-range policy proposal can be expected to have both significant political support and opposition. It would assure new revenues for the health sector through expanded insurance coverage. This should prove attractive to the hospital sector and certain groups of physicians, especially newly trained physicians. Primary care physicians should welcome the new physician payment reform, but it could prove threatening to surgeons and other specialty physicians. It should receive support from consumer groups and labor. Small businesses may be concerned by the new proposed administrative and financial burdens. The insurance industry should be supportive of expanded employer plan coverage but may oppose Medicaid expansion for those above the poverty level. Recognition of the problems of the uninsured, poor children and women, and the elderly needing long-term care is growing and should increase broad public support.

The political feasibility of the proposal could be expanded by a phased implementation of the proposal. Small steps in each of the features could be taken, and experience with these provisions obtained before moving on to the next phase. For example, it is possible to begin by expanding Medicaid coverage for those up to 75 percent of the poverty level, followed by those up to 100 percent of the poverty level, followed by the relaxation of the assets test. Long-term care coverage could begin with home health benefit coverage expansions, followed by nursing home coverage. Employer plan standards could start with larger firms or with smaller employer premium contributions. Provider payment reform provisions could be phased in gradually, gaining experience with each successive round of legislation.

It is extremely desirable, however, that such a phased-in approach move each component of the proposal forward in each phase. Otherwise politically popular elements will be enacted first with no action on the more controversial elements.

A long-range policy proposal, regardless of its ultimate shape, would greatly improve the health policy deliberation process. The current system of relying on year-to-year changes in health financing programs without any consensus on a longer range plan leads to gimmickry and instability in the health system. It gives undue weight to the fiscal objective of cutting budgetary outlays rather than basing health policy on social goals to be achieved by the health sector. I hope that my long-range policy proposal will facilitate informed debate leading to such a consensus.

REFERENCES

Further details on many of the elements of the long-range policy proposal presented here may be found in the following sources:

Davis, Karen, and Diane Rowland. *Medicare Policy: New Directions for Health and Long-Term Care.* Baltimore: Johns Hopkins Press, 1986.

_____, Gerard Anderson, Steven Renn, Diane Rowland, Carl Schramm, and Earl Steinberg. "Health Care Cost Containment: Lessons from the Past and Options for the Future." Draft manuscript, 1986.

_____. "Medicaid: MediGap Coverage for the Poor Elderly." Testimony before the Subcommittee on Health and the Environment, Committee on Energy and Commerce, U.S. House of Representatives, March 1986.

U.S. Department of Health and Human Services. Office of the Assistant Secretary for Planning and Evaluation. *National Health Plan Working Papers.* Vols. 1 and 2. January 1981.

2

TOWARD A MODEL SYSTEM FOR THE FINANCING AND DELIVERY OF HEALTH CARE IN THE UNITED STATES

Alain C. Enthoven

OVERVIEW

I believe that the United States ought to move promptly and decisively to a system of *universal, comprehensive* coverage of health care services in a system that is designed to seek both economic efficiency and justice. I believe that such a system could be both administratively and fiscally practical in today's context, though I recognize that there are formidable political obstacles based on both entrenched self-interest and widespread lack of understanding of the situation.

In many ways our society recognizes that nobody should be denied needed health services because of an inability to pay and that nobody should be subjected to extreme financial hardship because of illness. We have Medicare, Medicaid, tax-subsidized employer-paid coverage, numerous special programs, and public providers of last resort. When a seriously ill person is denied care by a hospital, there is widespread indignation and sometimes passage of an "antidumping" law. The gaps in coverage are arbitrary and indefensible. While I can explain the system in terms of historical evolution and the interplay of interest groups, I am convinced that there can be no rational defense of a system that denies coverage to a widow who has had cancer while granting large tax subsidies for comprehensive health coverage to an employed executive.

By *universal* I mean that every person would be offered the opportunity to enroll in a health care financing and delivery organization at a cost that is reasonable in relation to family income. As a rough indication of what I mean, I suggest a federal subsidy toward each person's coverage equal to 40 percent of the cost of an efficient plan. A higher pecentage would be desirable if resources were available. In the case of people with incomes below the poverty line, federal and state subsidies should pay the full cost. Between the poverty line and twice that level, a sliding-scale should apply so that nobody loses coverage or faces a large "notch" in the cost of coverage. (I recognize that present economic and political conditions might only support less generous subsidies.)

There always will be some people whose personal lifestyles or habits will not be compatible with signing up for health care coverage and carrying a membership card. Others may attempt to take a free ride and not make their premium contributions. The system can and should be designed with incentives to discourage this behavior. Although there will always be a need for a system of public providers of last resort, our society should seek to minimize the number of people dependent on it.

The model system I propose would generalize to the whole population the kind of system that serves Stanford University employees and other employees who have multiple-choice health plan arrangements.

By *comprehensive* I mean essentially the list of services termed Basic Health Services in the HMO Act. (One can argue about some of the details. Should the number of covered acute mental health visits be twenty, or ten, or thirty? I consider those questions to be minor details for present purposes.) Moreover, I believe these services should be covered with a minimum of deductibles, copays, and coinsurance. Providers control the overwhelming majority of costs. The system should be structured to encourage consumers to choose economical systems and to encourage providers to organize and deliver services economically.

The system should be designed to seek both justice and economic efficiency. I believe these can be reconciled to a reasonable degree. Some of the elements of a good model of how to do this are in Section 1876 of the Medicare Law. (However, in my 1986 paper on managed competition, I noted some important deficiencies in the design of Section 1876.) Each beneficiary is categorized by medical risk, and the Medicare program makes a contribution to the Health Maintenance Organization or Competitive Medical Plan (HMO/CMP) of the beneficiary's choice that is proportional to expected medical costs in that person's category. Thus, the sixty-five-year-old and the eighty-five-year-old pay the same dues to the same HMO, but the government contributes much more on behalf of the latter. Incentives for efficiency are built in because the government's contribution is in a fixed dollar amount so that beneficiaries who join a more costly system pay the extra costs themselves and are thus motivated to consider carefully the value for their money.

I believe the system should be *decentralized* and *pluralistic*. The health care system of the United States cannot possibly be run from Washington. Centralized European systems are extremely rigid and resistant to badly needed innovation. Moreover, they tend to become politicized. The national program should accommodate a wide variety of systems and styles of care to accommodate a variety of patient and provider preferences.

Finally, the national system should be consumer-driven. The present U.S. health care system has been built by and for providers with little or no incentive to give consumers value for money. I have expressed my belief by calling my proposal for universal health insurance the Consumer Choice Health Plan (Enthoven, *Consumer Choice*, 1978; 1980). The driving force should be consumer preferences. The government cannot compel good service willingly, kindly, and cheerfully provided. But in a suitably structured competitive market system, the health care plans that figure out how to do this will be the survivors. In other words, a rational and satisfactory health care financing and delivery policy will make high-quality care and service—as well as economy—in every provider's interest.

BASIC PRINCIPLES

The model system I propose would generalize to the whole population the kind of system that serves Stanford University employees and other employees who have multiple-choice health plan arrangements. Each November, Stanford employees are presented with a menu of choices for the coming year and a substantial fixed dollar contribution by the University, usable only as part payment toward one of the contracting coverages. The menu of choice includes several Health Maintenance Organizations (HMOs) and one Preferred Provider Insurance scheme. We have abandoned as obsolete our traditional indemnity insurance plan.

In the model system, every plan would cover a benefit package at least as comprehensive as Basic Health Services under the HMO Act. (This is not to argue against more extensive mental health coverage; it is to argue that we begin with a solid but financially realistic floor.) Copayments would be in defined, finite amounts that consumers could understand in advance (e.g., "$10 per office visit," and not unintelligible formulas such as "insurance pays 80 percent of UCR"). And they would be limited in aggregate annual amount as they are under the HMO Act.

To clarify my proposal, let me contrast the concepts of my model system with the principles of the "medical guild" that have dominated health care finance in this country to date.

The economic principles of the medical guild are as follows:

(a) *Free choice of provider.* For providers, this means that every provider can participate in every insurance scheme on equal terms. The purpose and the effect of this is to prevent economic competition and cost consciousness on the demand side. The insured patient isn't cost conscious because treatment is covered by insurance; the payor can't control cost because it has no bargaining power. The patient's free choice of provider means the payor (usually the insurance company) doesn't have the power to direct patients away from high-cost providers. In the context of fairly comprehensive insurance, free choice of provider, or "Guild Free Choice" as Charles Weller (1984) called it, is a blank check for providers. (I will explain what I consider to be the appropriate interpretation of freedom below.)

(b) *Free choice of prescription without interference by a third party.* This principle permits what economists call "provider-induced demand." The doctor who profits from providing the services is the one who recommends or prescribes them. This principle has been invoked to block the development of utilization review and quality control.

(c) *Direct understanding between doctor and patient regarding fees, with no contracting with a third party.* This exploits to the maximum the obvious vulnerability of the sick patient and the family. How many people are going to try to drive a hard bargain or question the need for services for their seriously ill family member? This principle also means that there is no connection between the doctor and the insurer, so the patient is left not knowing what the insurance really buys. In addition, the doctor does not have to deal with an informed purchaser who has bargaining power.

(d) *Solo practice as a way of better preserving a seamless web of mutual coercion.* Within a large multispecialty group practice, physicians could refer among themselves and thus, as a group, become an economic competitor.

These principles can be contrasted with a model system made up of Competitive Medical Plans (CMPs), based on the following principles. (I use the term CMP here, not in its legal sense as defined in Section 1876 of the Medicare Law, but rather as a generic term that includes HMOs and at least some Preferred Provider Insurance [PPI] schemes.)

(a) *Market free choice.* The patient voluntarily accepts a choice of providers limited to those contracting with the CMP of his or her choice, usually for a year at a time. Thus, the patient contracts in advance for whatever comprehensive health care services he or she may need.

(b) *Physician practice is subject to peer review for quality and economy.* The contracting physicians accept responsibility to provide care for all members of the enrolled population.

(c) *Premiums are paid directly to the organization that provides or organizes and contracts for the care, in the form of periodic payments set in advance.* This gives the provider organization a fixed prospective budget and a defined population for which it is responsible. This gives it the opportunity and incentive to allocate and manage resources efficiently.

(d) *Formally or informally, a CMP involves some form of collaborative effort among physicians from the full range of specialties.*

The model system could include PPI schemes organized and operated by insurance companies, provided that a sufficient number and distribution (by geography and specialty) of providers are available to serve the enrolled population so that enrollees could reasonably expect to get all their care from contracting providers if they wanted to. I have not figured out how to encode this in a legal definition. But I expect, with the growth of HMOs, that market forces will eventually take care of the PPI schemes that do not have enough preferred providers to do the job.

Basically, I look forward to the euthanasia of the indemnity-insurance model, in which the patient has no way of knowing or controlling the cost of care for an illness. This would occur as a result of free choices by cost-conscious consumers.

Finally, the model system I propose would be administratively simple from the point of view of the patient. The present Medicare system—which is a direct product of the "medical guild"—is nothing short of a monstrosity from this point of view. Picture the plight of the elderly couple, one of whom is seriously ill in the hospital. Assume they are fortunate enough to have some sort of supplemental insurance. Let me assume the husband is sick and the wife wants to focus her attention on caring for her spouse. The attending physician calls upon a procession of "_____ologists," each of whom comes to the hospital for a series of tests and visits. Soon the wife finds her mailbox filled with complicated bills, all due in thirty days, sometimes accompanied by various threats if not paid promptly. "You are responsible for paying the balance shown within thirty days." She gets a Medicare claim form and sends the bills to Medicare. Several months later she receives a check and a complicated statement explaining why Medicare is paying perhaps half the bills. Medicare may refuse to pay some because of lack of information or because Medicare's fiscal intermediary disagrees with her husband's doctors about what care is appropriate. So she calls the hospital for the information. Then she repeats the process with her supplemental insurance company. Eventually she discovers that what she thought was fairly comprehensive insurance has large "air pockets."

Contrast that with the situation of a similar couple who belongs to an HMO on a risk-basis contract with Medicare. They pay a modest monthly premium that is fixed in advance, predictable, and easy to understand. For the comprehensive covered services they receive from the HMO, *they get no bill*. It is all prepaid. They exercised their cost consciousness in their annual choice of plan. I believe the savings in social cost from this system are large.

Competition

The system I have proposed has often been characterized as competitive, and that is one of its most prominent features, though far from the whole story. At the broadest level of generality, a system of economic competition of alternative health care financing and delivery plans can be described in terms of four principles.

The first is *periodic choice*. Once a year, each person or family would be offered the opportunity to join one of several competing health care financing and delivery plans. People who are not satisfied with the service or care they receive can switch at the next enrollment. Government would assure each person the opportunity to enroll at a reasonable price. The pattern of annual enrollment for a year at a time has worked well in the market for millions of employees for many years. It is supplemented by the HMOs' grievance procedures and the possibility of appeal to the employee benefits office to resolve the problems of those very few people who feel they have made a mistake and want to change before the year is over.

The second is *cost conscious choice through fixed-dollar subsidies.* Each person's premium is subsidized, but the subsidy is in a fixed dollar amount independent of choice plan. This is to motivate cost consciousness. The person who chooses a plan that costs, say, twenty dollars per month must pay that amount out of his or her own net after-tax income. That motivates him or her to seek value for money, and it puts the health plans under economic pressure to produce value for money.

The third principle is *equal rules for all competitors.* There cannot be a "free market" in health insurance. A "free market" is subject to extreme market failure. Insurers don't want to insure the sick who need coverage. And the well don't want to buy coverage that subsidizes the sick. We have about 35 million Americans in the "free market" sector of our health insurance economy; they have no coverage. The market for health care coverage is not naturally competitive. A competitive market in health insurance can only work if it is governed by carefully drawn rules that must apply equally to all competitors. *Thus, I am recommending a model based on a careful design, not just on any old thing called "competition."* In particular, the U.S. health care economy today is decidedly not "competitive" in that sense.

The fourth principle is that, generally speaking, through CMPs, *the providers in any community are divided up into competing economic units.*

Managed Competition

Many proponents and critics of the competition idea share the misconception that competition means a market made up of health care financing and delivery plans on the supply side and individual consumers on the demand side, without a carefully drawn set of rules designed to mitigate the effects of the market failures endemic to health care financing and delivery and without mediation by some form of collective action on the demand side. Some see it as just one more field for the operation of Adam Smith's "invisible hand." That isn't the idea at all. Such a market does not and cannot work. Health insurance and health care markets are not naturally competitive. Health insurance markets are vulnerable to many failures that result from attempts by insurers to select risks, segment markets, and protect themselves from "free riders" who seek to postpone buying insurance until they get sick.

Yet we have seen several large-scale and long-term examples in which a sponsoring organization has organized and managed a reasonably successful competitive market system to serve its beneficiary population. I am referring, for example, to the Federal Employees Health Benefits

Program, the similar California State Public Employees Retirement System, and the programs of Stanford University and the University of California. (The design of these systems is far from perfect, in my view, but they have served their beneficiaries well for a long time.) What these experiences show is that the correct concept of the competition that can work is "managed competition," in which intelligent active agents on the demand side contract with the health care plans and continuously structure and adjust the market to overcome attempts to avoid price competition. I call these agents "sponsors." A sponsor is an agency that assures the members of a defined population group the opportunity to buy health care coverage. The sponsor also subsidizes the beneficiaries' purchases to discourage free riders and to achieve equity. The sponsor for Medicare beneficiaries is the *Health Care Financing Administration.*

How Will the System Be Financed?

Everybody hates taxes these days, and a forthright answer to this question is bound to alienate many readers and draw many denunciations from politicians.

I do not have a complete and precise plan, but I do have some ideas that I consider relevant and important.

First, the subsidies to everyone's health insurance would obviously have to be tax supported.

Second, in general I favor very broadly based taxes, such as payroll and "flat" income taxes, with few or no exclusions, so as to permit low rates and to minimize economic distortion. Thus, I believe that a significant part of the subsidies should be financed by general revenues.

Third, I believe that Medicare should and will continue to be payroll-tax financed (Part A). I believe it would be appropriate to relate the Part B contribution to income. That is, instead of paying about one-quarter of the cost of Part B, leaving the rest to be paid out of general revenues, beneficiaries with incomes at twice the poverty line or more should be required to contribute a modest amount, such as 1 or 2 percent of the excess of their adjusted gross incomes over twice the poverty line, until their contribution equals the average per-beneficiary cost of Part B. There are many financially secure retired people for whom this would be no hardship. If there are any gaps left, I would favor making Medicare coverage and payroll taxes absolutely universal for people over sixty-five not covered by a comparable program.

Fourth, the most important "new source" of revenue I propose would actually be a restructuring of existing subsidies. I have recently estimated that the exclusion of employer contributions from the incomes of employees subject to income and payroll taxes cost the federal budget a potential $50 billion in 1986. ("Potential" because the actual revenue loss depends on how quickly employers and individuals move to take advantage of tax breaks [Enthoven 1985].) This tax break for employer-provided health insurance is a powerful subsidy to health insurance purchases. I have criticized it on four grounds (Enthoven 1984). First, the cost to the federal budget is very large and growing very rapidly. In the 1970s, the cost to the budget doubled its share of GNP in a decade. Second, the distribution of the subsidy is very inequitable. In 1983, the Congressional Budget Office estimated the subsidy was worth $83 to a household with an income of $10,000 to $15,000 and $622 to a household with an income of $50,000 to $100,000. It was worth nothing to people without employer contributions. If the justification of the subsidy is to respond to need or to encourage purchase of health insurance, its relationship to income should be opposite—that is, greater for people with low incomes and without jobs. Third, by subsidizing the marginal cost of health coverage purchases, it encourages upper-income employed people to buy more costly coverages, thus exacerbating the cost-increasing incentives in the system. And fourth, it reinforces the link between jobs and health insurance. People lose an important subsidy when they lose their jobs—arguably when they need it most.

For the same cost to the federal budget, it would be possible to offer everybody a subsidy to their health insurance purchase equal to 40 percent of their premium cost up to a limit on subsidized premiums of $65 per individual per month, $130 per couple, and $195 per family.

In the spring of 1986, Senator Durenberger introduced Senate Bill 2485, which would repeal the exclusion and replace it with such a subsidy (U.S. Congress 1986). The amounts of subsidy were computed to produce "budget neutrality," but larger subsidies would be desirable if resources were available.

By lowering the top marginal tax rates, the recent Tax Reform Act reduced the revenue loss associated with the exclusion. The average federal marginal tax rate (income and payroll taxes) will drop from about 35 percent to 30 percent. The revenue loss for 1987 and beyond needs to be reestimated under the new conditions. But it will still be a large sum of money. Moreover, since states conform to the federal definition of income in this respect, they too lose large amounts of revenue to this cause.

If the federal government were to subsidize 40 percent of premium costs, it would become a much more manageable proposition for states to subsidize a large part of the rest for poor people.

How might states raise money for this? I have a few modest suggestions. First, repeal of the exclusion of employer contributions from taxable incomes would generate a new revenue source. States under constitutional spending limits like California could characterize the subsidy as a refundable tax credit usable only as a premium contribution to a qualified health plan. That would make it "tax reduction" instead of "public spending." Second, as more people became insured, states and counties could reduce their net outlays on public hospitals. Third, universal coverage would, in my view, bring important efficiency gains. Fourth, I favor an increased federal excise tax on tobacco and alcohol equal in revenues to the actuarially estimated cost that abuse of these substances causes to the health care system. The tax should be federal to make it harder to evade, but the proceeds should be used to subsidize health care coverage. This tax is justified by the "free market" principle that those who generate social costs by voluntary behavior should have to pay them.

Finally, I believe serious consideration should be given to a payroll and self-employment tax payable by employers who do not provide their employees with health insurance, with the proceeds to be used to subsidize health insurance purchases by the otherwise uninsured. This would make health insurance contributions mandatory.

How Will Quality of Care Be Monitored and Controlled?

This is an exceedingly important issue. Space permits only an outline of an answer.

First, there is an appalling lack of quality assurance in American medicine. Many doctors seem to think it has something to do with fee-for-service or the prestige of their residency programs. Organized medicine has systematically resisted quality assurance. Only recently have government and employers begun to require some sort of quality review, and that is in its infancy.

I visualize several approaches to the quality problem, some of which are inherent in the managed-competition concept, some of which are complementary to it.

The dominant fee-for-service solo practice system breeds and rewards bad-quality medicine. It actually rewards providers with more money for errors. Picture the poor, seriously ill hospitalized patient. The attending physician calls in some "___ologist" for a consultation. If the consultant makes a shrewd and accurate diagnosis on the first visit, suggests just the right therapy to the attending physician (which deals effectively with the problem), and bows out, he or she will be paid for one consultation and will pass up the opportunity to make a lot of money. In the alternative, the consultant might fail to diagnose the problem, try this and that unsuccessfully, order a bunch of tests, make repeated visits, and be paid hundreds of dollars for not much work. The attending physician doesn't want to control the spending of the consultant because he or she wants to be called as a consultant on the other doctor's case. The solo practice system works against peer review. If the peers take action against a poor performer, they may be seen as threatening an economic competitor for monopolistic goals. The system motivates doctors to hold onto patients inappropriately when they should refer.

I do not want to suggest that prepaid group practice (PGP) is perfect. But I believe that in the long run, variations on that model will be the winners in a competitive process. And I see in that model many quality-enhancing dynamics. Quality and economy usually go hand in hand. The right diagnosis made promptly, followed by the appropriate procedure done by a most proficient specialist, is best for quality and economy. The doctors in PGPs do best if they do it right the first time. They pay for their mistakes. If a surgeon botches an operation—necessitating a prolonged hospital stay and reoperation—in the HMO format, the doctors pay for it; they don't make money off it. That motivates them to put surgery in the hands of proficient surgeons. There is built-in peer review because there is shared risk and responsibility. The doctor who sees his or her partner perform poorly has a powerful incentive, a right, and an organizational structure within which to press for corrective action.

So in the model system I envisage, increasingly cohesive health care organizations will have incentives to improve quality for the sake of their reputations and economy.

Some aspects of quality of care and service can be judged adequately by individual patients and their families. But some very important aspects, such as whether effective medical care makes sick patients better, are statistical matters that can only be judged on the experience of large populations. This is a very undeveloped area, but one in which large sponsors have a much better chance than unaffiliated individuals to develop or obtain the data to evaluate quality.

I believe that there ought to be state-mandated reporting on all hospital cases with data sufficient to support the development of sophisticated systems of risk-adjusted monitoring of outcomes (Blumberg 1986.) For example, for coronary artery bypass surgery, all risk factors considered, is this team's thirty-day survival rate better or worse than par?

This type of analysis has a very long way to go. Concerned citizens—such as those represented by AARP—should press hard for public support of it.

In addition, Medicare beneficiaries in each community should band together to collect and publish evaluative information on CMPs of the sort that is published in *Consumer Reports*. Better information and quality consciousness are keys to forcing CMPs to improve quality of care.

Who Are the Key Decision Makers? What Are Their Roles?

The most important decision makers in the model system I propose are *consumers*. They would make cost-conscious, increasingly informed choices of CMPs. If satisfied, they would stay with their plan and tell their friends. If dissatisfied, they would "vote with their feet."

In a decentralized, competitive private market system, health plans must respond to consumer preferences to survive. Centralized government-controlled systems respond to provider preferences. The reason for this is not hard to find. People diversify in consumption but specialize in production. Thus, they are much more likely to vote and contribute on behalf of their well-focused producer interest than their diffuse consumer interest. A rise in the price of milk is a minor issue for a typical family but a life and death matter for a dairy farmer. Two of the most prominent features of the British National Health Service are provider domination and a low level of service to patients (long waiting lines, insensitive scheduling practices, inconvenient hours, etc.) (Enthoven, *Reflections on the Management*, 1985). And there is nothing the British voters can do about it. (The most articulate opt out into the private sector if they have the money.)

The next-most-important decision makers are the sponsors who contract with health plans and structure the choices presented to their sponsored populations. The sponsors are large employers, employer coalitions, some unions, and government agencies such as the Health Care Financing Administration. The role of sponsors is spelled out in some detail in my paper on managed competition (Enthoven 1986). In a system of universal coverage, I envisage state agencies acting as sponsors for the otherwise unsponsored. The federal government would be the principal subsidizer and would set the general rules for the competitive market system.

The role of providers would be to learn to organize and manage high-quality cost-effective care in a manner that is efficient and satisfying to consumers.

How Will Cost Be Controlled?

Cost will be controlled by each CMP as a part of its competitive effort to attract the membership of cost-conscious consumers.

In the model system I recommend, the emphasis is on a considered, cost-conscious annual choice of health plan and not on cost consciousness at the point of medical need. When my injured child is lying bleeding on the operating table is not the time when I want to begin negotiating with the doctor about fees or the number of sutures needed.

The system I recommend puts maximum pressure on providers to organize the system efficiently. This is appropriate because the overwhelming majority of cost-generating decisions (weighted by dollar volume) are made by providers, not consumers. The great majority of costs are for the care of very sick people. Their care is in the hands of providers.

My main reason for optimism that this will work is the experience of group-practice HMOs. For example, in its Health Insurance Experiment, the RAND Corporation found that patients cared for in Seattle by Group Health Cooperative of Puget Sound (GHCPS) had a 40 percent lower hospitalization rate and consumed 28 percent fewer resources overall, compared with similar people (stratified random sample) under the insured fee-for-service system. And GHCPS did this in the absence of significant competition from other cost-effective systems. In my judgment, under serious competitive pressure, it would be possible for them to make substantial improvements in efficiency. (In my experience as an industrial manager, I found there was nothing like a serious competitive threat to motivate the workforce to improve efficiency.)

Starting with the present, extremely wasteful system, there are many ways to cut costs substantially while improving the quality of care. Only a few are (a) appropriate physician incentives; (b) serious quality assurance, including risk-adjusted monitoring of outcomes; (c) careful matching of resources used to the needs of the population served (surgeons with full operating schedules are better for economy and quality); (d) regional concentration of complex, specialized services such as open-heart surgery; (e) evaluated choice and use of new technology; and (f) elimination of vast amounts of paperwork by eliminating billing and collecting for individual items of service (Enthoven, *Shattuck Lecture*, 1978).

Cost-effectiveness and systematic decision analysis applied to medical care is in its infancy. I teach a course on the subject and have found few worthwhile readings published before 1980. There is an enormous potential for more rational, evaluated medical practice, but it will take organization and powerful competitive pressures to move the system. This is admittedly a long-term strategy. But the promises of quick fixes for the problem of rapidly growing health expenditures are false.

How Comprehensive Is the System in Terms of Access to Care and Scope of Coverage?

The system I am describing would cover all active medical care—physicians' services, acute hospital care, lab work, X rays, etc.—generally as defined in the HMO Act. (I am not unalterably committed to all the details of the HMO Act's definition. I simply consider it a useful definition or example of comprehensive care.)

The two most significant omissions from this are long-term inpatient and outpatient psychiatric care and long-term care. In the case of the former, I believe that (1) as a matter of priority, making coverage of medical care as defined in the HMO Act universal is more important; and (2) the definition and cost control of mental health benefits need more study. I will comment on long-term care in a later section.

Access to services would and should be as it is in those areas where HMOs compete vigorously. HMOs provide or arrange services, as needed, twenty-four hours a day and seven days a week.

With respect to geographic access, the traditional guild system has worsened geographic distribution by providing open-ended subsidies to care in wealthy, attractive areas where doctors like to live, while failing to provide steady medical purchasing power in less attractive, poorer areas. My proposals would change this. I believe the predictable consequence of this would be a gradual reduction in the number of physicians per capita in places like San Francisco and Boston and an increase in underserved areas where they are needed. The result would be a more equitable distribution.

As a practical matter, I believe that if the financial incentives are corrected and made equitable, market forces will produce about as good a geographic distribution of physicians as can be achieved. Certainly direct government efforts to alter the geographic distribution, in this country and others, have not been successful.

What Will the Delivery System Look Like?

I would expect the delivery system to look pretty much the way it does in areas such as Minneapolis-Saint Paul, where several HMOs compete vigorously and serve a large proportion of the population. Under the system of incentives I propose, the competition would be even more intense because there would no longer be a subsidized "open-ended sector" in which cost-unconscious providers could find refuge.

There would be a significant variety in terms of systems and styles of care, in accordance with the preferences of consumers and providers. There would be multispecialty group practices, many of which would find a balance between large centers for specialty care and primary care satellites for convenience. There would be Independent Practice Associations (IPAs) and a variety of network models. By and large, the physical appearance and apparent practice styles would not change much, except for changes that would improve geographic and temporal access. (It is clear in Minneapolis-Saint Paul and in the midpeninsula area where I live that HMOs compete on access.) Many would be covered under Preferred Provider Insurance (PPI), and HMOs would adopt PPI features. There would continue to be fee-for-service practitioners. I would expect the CMPs to experiment with and "empirically tune" payment systems to reward physician productivity and ability to attract patients. But there would be few fee-for-service practitioners in the traditional guild sense— that is, unconstrained by any contracts with CMPs. We will see fee-for-service only in the context of "contract medicine," i.e., based on fees and utilization controls negotiated in advance.

I expect there would always be a few renowned specialists and a few primary care physicians catering to the carriage trade who would practice outside the system, as occurs in the United Kingdom. For practical purposes, however, this would not be important.

Would there still be proprietary institutions? The distinction between for-profit and not-for-profit is now blurred. I doubt that the investor-owned hospital chains will grow much in the next decade because hospitals are in excess supply and will be forced to sell services at marginal cost that is below average cost. They will, therefore, not make the profits needed to finance expansion.

I believe the economic performance of the investor-owneds and those similarly situated and the not-for-profits has not been very different. I see no persuasive evidence to support the proposition that the for-profits are more efficient. To me the most important differences between the two are in the areas of public policy advocacy and corporate culture. The investor-owned hospitals and the commercial insurance companies, alongside organized medicine, lobby intensively to protect their right to make a profit. I believe the nonprofit hospital organizations and HMOs are much more concerned with promoting public policies that will assure widespread access to care. Personally, I would like to see the values espoused by the nonprofit sector predominate, but I see nothing to be gained by trying to legislate against for-profit companies.

How Will Long-Term Care Be Financed and Delivered?

I have not studied the problems of long-term care in any depth, so I would prefer to say little or nothing on this subject. Let me offer just a few general ideas. Our present system of financing is a scandal. The taxpayers end up paying for about half of nursing home care, but first many people are forced to "spend down" into poverty so that they can qualify for Medicaid. Family savings are wiped out. Devoted couples in long-term marriages are forced to consider divorce so that the one partner will not be impoverished when the other must be confined in a nursing home. This system is cruel and irrational and cries out for reform.

I believe that studies and experiments concerning strictly private-sector approaches to financing are commendable and well-intentioned. But I believe they are bound to fail. A typical insurance scheme would ask me to start contributing now, at age fifty-six, for a service that I might need twenty-five or thirty years from now. I do not believe it would be possible to design a satisfactory contract. How does one define a nursing home or need for long-term care thirty years from now? How much will services cost? Who decides what I "need"? The problems of risk selection (people with histories of heart problems do not expect to survive that long so they do not buy insurance), moral hazard (I paid for it so I want it even if you think I do not need it), and general vagueness and uncertainty about the service are insuperable. This market is even more prone to failure than the market for insurance for acute care. The fact that long-term care insurance in the private sector is virtually nonexistent is evidence for this conclusion.

I believe we need a universal, mandatory social insurance program to cover long-term care. Half of it could be paid for by diverting the Medicaid funds now used for that purpose. The other half might be paid for in part by diverting Social Security pension funds to this purpose. One mechanism for doing this might be simply to declare all Social Security pension payments a part of the recipient's taxable income and use the proceeds for this purpose. (I can imagine the political difficulties, and responsible leadership is needed. I do not believe that increasing the flow of subsidies from the working population to the retired population is economically or politically realistic.) After a substantial deductible the insurance would cover most of the nursing home cost in excess of an estimated average cost of living if the patient were not institutionalized. But there are serious problems of incentives in a traditional insurance-entitlement scheme. Creating a universal entitlement to free nursing home care could tip the balance for many families in favor of institutionalization of someone they now care for at home. So a great deal of care must go into how such a program is designed.

With respect to the organization and delivery of long-term care services, we need a framework that encourages a continuing process of innovation, especially in alternatives to institutionalization. We need to get away from entitlements to institutionalization combined with little or no support for those who would avoid it. Above all, we should avoid a system that freezes the present system of care in place. The spirit of what I am proposing for medical care is much the same as the spirit that motivates the "Social HMO" experiments now underway. I favor lots of Social HMO experiments in order to develop the concepts and methods for integrating services in such a way as to support frail elderly in their familiar noninstitutional settings.

The evolution of Social HMOs would be a natural complement to the medical system reforms I recommend. In fact, the HMOs I recommend could form an organizational base for such a development.

I believe we need a universal, mandatory social insurance program to cover long-term care. Half of it could be paid for by diverting the Medicaid funds now used for that purpose. The other half might be paid for in part by diverting Social Security pension funds to this purpose.

What Role for Medicare and Medicaid?

The Medicare program would continue as the sponsor agency for all Medicare-eligibles. However, the traditional Medicare insurance program, which is based on the "guild free choice" model, would gradually be replaced by the capitation-financed model described in Section 1876. When sufficient HMO capacity is available in each service area, I recommend that new beneficiaries be required to select a CMP. The traditional model should be phased out, just as we have done at Stanford.

Here is what I wrote in my 1986 article on managed competition:

> To get the most health care for the beneficiaries from the available funds, HCFA's role needs to be recast from managing an insurance program to sponsoring beneficiaries in a competitive market. . . . HCFA's procedures should be modelled on successful designs in the FEHBP and the private sector. For example, in each market area there should be a single, coordinated, open enrollment managed and run by HCFA or a local broker agency contracting with HCFA. (I am thinking, for example, of Health Choice in Portland, Oregon.) HCFA should produce or contract to have

produced useful information for consumers. Communities and senior citizens' groups should become involved.

I hope to see the Medicaid program completely replaced by the program of federal–state subsidies I have described and the state "sponsor for the unsponsored" agencies.

The approach I have outlined would offer some large advantages to Medicaid beneficiaries and other poor people. First, it would buy their way into membership in the CMPs that serve employed middle-income people. Thus, it would be an important step toward the mainstream ideal. Second, they would be enrolled as regular dues-paying members, not stigmatized as welfare recipients. Third, membership and coverage would be continuous; it would not fluctuate with income or other variables determining eligibility. Finally, in the universal system I advocate, all the poor would be covered, not just those in the welfare categories. Large savings could be achieved by elimination of the eligibility-determination process and the administrative burdens resulting from discontinuity of coverage that, in turn, is the result of fluctuating eligibility.

Why Retired People Should Favor the CMP or "Competing HMO" Model

I believe there are several powerful reasons why retired people—in their own self-interest—should favor the competitive model I have described.

First, it is and will become increasingly important that we organize the medical care system for maximum efficiency. The financing of health care for the aged will be increasingly caught in a bind created by the cost-increasing forces of advancing medical technology and longevity on the one hand and taxpayer resistance and the dwindling number of active workers per retiree on the other. The situation will be extremely tight. There just is not some easy source of money.

Experience with HMOs so far demonstrates substantial potential for efficiency gains. I believe that if the incentives of the total system were reformed, efficiency gains could be even greater than we have seen so far and factor prices could be driven down to competitive levels.

The only way known to man to achieve efficiency on a sustained basis is through cost-conscious competition. The British National Health Service limits spending (and holds down factor prices very effectively) but it clearly does not produce care efficiently. The Canadian fee-for-service system does not organize care efficiently either.

Second, retired people especially need an *organized system* of care, a system that integrates inpatient and outpatient care, a system that stays with you when you leave the hospital and doesn't dump you into a "no-care zone," a system that accepts responsibility for organizing and financing total care. I believe HMO-like organizations are our only hope for that.

Third, the HMO format creates total financial predictability for the cost of covered services. And it leaves the patient and family with no unexpected cash-flow problems (while Medicare may take three months and the supplemental insurer another two months to pay). All HMO providers accept assignment.

Fourth, the HMO can and, at least in the prepaid group practice (PGP) models, does eliminate vast amounts of complex and burdensome paperwork. In the HMO, other than some nominal copayments, the patient receives no bills for covered services.

In the face of these advantages, I know that some people will still allege significant disadvantages. One of the most significant limitations is that some more educated and more affluent people really will value the freedom to go outside the HMO anytime they want if they have a serious problem. "If I'm really sick, I want to be able to go to Stanford." Of course people who want that freedom should have it, but they should pay what it costs. I believe that hybrid HMO-PPI models are already evolving to accommodate this desire. That is the beauty of market approaches.

A related problem concerns the "snow birds." Some people like to spend the summers at home in Minnesota and the winters in Florida. Again, I think the market will accommodate this. Preferred Provider Insurance hybrids may do it. If beneficiaries winter and summer in two areas served by the same national HMO organization or PPI plan, that system will accommodate them nicely. Some HMOs have formed reciprocal arrangements for this purpose.

Some people don't like "the HMO style." PPI and IPAs can take care of them. And the big HMOs are now trying to find ways of looking more personal, less institutional.

Another frequent objection is that it would take too long for the competitive model to become effective. In the late 1970s and early 1980s, the conventional wisdom was that HMO membership could grow no more than 10 percent per year, at which rate it would take well into the next century to get most people into HMOs. Since then the growth rate of HMOs has picked up to some 25 percent per year. In 1982, the California legislature passed AB3480, overturning the previous "guild free choice" law and authorizing preferred provider insurance. Since then, PPI enrollment has grown explosively in California and other states. With appropriate legislation, management by HCFA, and support by organizations like AARP, I believe that HMOs and PPI plans together could enroll several million Medicare beneficiaries a year. The Blues would, of course, be a major factor in this, as they are already in several states.

What about rural areas? The competition of organized systems has led some systems to create rural primary care outposts in which they support a doctor, financially and professionally, recognizing that he or she can be a source of referrals. The first requirement for rural areas is a steady flow of medical purchasing power, as would be created by my Consumer Choice Health Plan or enactment of the Durenberger Bill.

Finally, what about the recent International Medical Centers, Inc., (IMC) scandal in Florida or the similar prepaid health plan scandals that marked Governor Reagan's administration in California (U.S. General Accounting Office 1986; Goldberg 1975)? Is this concept especially vulnerable to fraud and abuse? It is important to judge this question in perspective and not to reject a valid concept because of a few blemishes on its implementation. To do so would be like rejecting democracy because of the Wedtech or Iran-Contra scandals. In fact, the record of the established HMOs that serve private-sector employers has been very good. The abuses have been associated with special purpose organizations created largely to serve Medicare and Medicaid populations, and not with the established HMOs. There are rip-offs and scandals all over the medical care system, especially in the fee-for-service sector. For example, in 1978, before there was any significant HMO contracting with HCFA, the Inspector General of the Department of Health, Education, and Welfare estimated there was over $4.5 billion of waste, fraud, and abuse in Medicare and Medicaid in fiscal year 1977, virtually all of it in fee-for-service medicine (U.S. Department of Health, Education, and Welfare 1978). HMOs and CMPs are far less susceptible to abuse than the solo practice system because they are organized, and have audited financial statements and formal management controls. Solo practitioners do not have such accountability. The most important errors in the IMC and prepaid health plan scandals arose from an inappropriate application of the "free market" philosophy of the Reagan administration. Reagan officials believed that the free market would sort out the good from the bad health plans. This might be true in the long run, but people are not willing to show such patience in the case of medical care. Somebody might get hurt before the long run comes about. That is one reason why active management by a sponsor in a managed competition model is needed.

Government, in the case of Medicare and Medicaid, or any other sponsor, must exercise active surveillance over whether the contractors are delivering the services they contracted to perform—just as in any business situation. And they must take prompt corrective action when things begin to go wrong.

In the fee-for-service solo practice model, the individual patient must judge the individual doctor without the help of other organizations or information other than what friends say. There are no checks and balances to promote quality and economy. That's about like a spectator who doesn't know much about baseball trying to judge the quality of a batter by watching one or two times at bat. In the managed-competition model, in addition to the individual patient judging the individual doctor, there is systematic peer review within organizations of doctors, and there are sponsors evaluating and judging the performance of competing organizations. For the baseball fan, it would also be like having the batting averages and the opinions of the baseball writers.

REFERENCES

Blumberg, M. "Risk-adjusting Health Care Outcomes: A Methodological Review." *Medical Care Review* 43(2): 351–96 (Fall 1986).

Enthoven, A. "Consumer Choice Health Plan." *New England Journal of Medicine* 298 (12 and 13): 650–58 and 709–20 (1978).

———. "Shattuck Lecture—Cutting Cost without Cutting the Quality of Care." *New England Journal of Medicine* 298: 1229–38 (1978).

———. *Health Plan: The Only Practical Solution to the Soaring Cost of Medical Care.* Reading, Mass.: Addison-Wesley, 1980.

———. "A New Proposal to Reform the Tax Treatment of Health Insurance." *Health Affairs* 3 (1): 21–39 (Spring 1984).

———. "Health Tax Policy Mismatch." *Health Affairs* 4 (4): 5–14 (Winter 1985).

———. "Reflections on the Management of the National Health Service." Miffield Provincial Hospitals Trust Occasional Paper No. 5, 1985.

———. "Managed Competition in Health Care and the Unfinished Agenda." *Health Care Financing Review.* 1986 Annual Supplement (December 1986).

Goldberg, V. P. "Some Emerging Problems of Prepaid Health Plans in the Medi-Cal System." *Policy Analysis* 1 (1): 55–68 (Winter 1975).

U.S. Congress. S. 2485. 99th Cong. 2d sess. Introduced May 1986 by D. Durenberger.

U.S. Department of Health, Education, and Welfare. Office of Inspector General. *Annual Report*. March 31, 1978.

U.S. General Accounting Office (GAO). *Medicare Issues Raised by Florida Health Maintenance Organization Demonstrations*. July 1986.

Weller, C. "Free Choice as a Restraint of Trade in American Health Care Delivery and Insurance." *Iowa Law Review* 69: 1351–91 (1984).

3

A COMMENTARY ON THE
PAPER PREPARED BY
ALAIN ENTHOVEN

Robert L. Kane

There is much to support in Professor Enthoven's proposal and some areas that require clarification and expansion. He has declared himself in favor of universal, comprehensive coverage of health care services. Essentially this means everyone has an opportunity to enroll in an organized program that offers a standard set of benefits (based on those defined as the basic health services in the HMO Act) at a price that would be subsidized at a rate equal to 40 percent of the cost of an efficient plan.

He has placed great faith in the prepaid practice system. I agree with his assessment that it is a great improvement over fee-for-service practice, but even with managed competition, it is not free from abuse. The solace he draws from the RAND experiment fails to recognize that such experiments demonstrate the best case but do not tell us much about what will happen in a less constrained environment.

He would use "managed competition" to minimize the need for other forces directed at the consumer such as deductibles, copays, and coinsurance. The recent report from the RAND health insurance experiment that showed a similar rate of inappropriate hospitalization among patients with and without copayments suggests that the reduced utilization produced by such devices may eliminate useful care. Since the RAND study specifically eliminated the elderly, the consequences for that group, which is more vulnerable to medical intervention, are likely more profound.

"Managed care" is a new term introduced to represent a more dynamic form of oversight and response to the American penchant for game playing. Enthoven is appropriately skeptical about the realism of fair competition in the medical marketplace and equally pessimistic about the ability of any staid set of rules to withstand provider manipulation.

He supports a decentralized and pluralistic system. Not surprisingly, he finds the ideal model in his own backyard. The heart of the Competitive Medical Plan (CMP) approach is a form of regulated competition with a sort of referee/commissioner overseeing the game. This individual (organization) is termed a "sponsor." The sponsor sets the rules (or interprets those produced by a higher central authority) and has the right to act on partial data to move expeditiously in what is importantly a dynamic system of regulation. The sponsor gathers data on the plan's performance and acts as a middleman with the consumer to prevent exploitation and to assure honest product representation.

In the less-regulated new world of medical competition, we have grown accustomed to the talk about market niches and tend to forget that they produce market chinks, which are usually left as the residual responsibility of the public sector (too often with the ironic accusation that such care is then less efficiently delivered than that provided privately).

Professor Enthoven indicates that the best way to assure fair competition is to insist that the competition be based on services rather than price. He is thus uncomfortable with the idea of high- and low-option plans, for example. He notes, too, that it is hard for consumers to judge the technical quality of care because the majority do not undergo major episodes of care frequently enough to gain the requisite experience. His health sponsors are thus in a much better position to note providers' batting averages and to monitor such important items as the health status of the sponsored population, treatments and risk-adjusted outcomes, hospital use by diagnosis, physician-encounter data, and who disenrolls and why.

ENTHOVEN'S COMPETITIVE SYSTEM

The heart of this proposal remains a competitive system, albeit within some constraints. In this model, the world would look something like the Twin Cities or Palo Alto, with a series of organized firms contracting to provide a predetermined package of services to enrollees. (It is interesting to note that in the list of successful models of managed care he includes the Federal Employees Health Benefits Program, a similar program in California, and those at Stanford and the University of California, but he makes no reference to the AHCSS program in Arizona, which was designed primarily for the indigent and which demonstrates some of the problems such a system can encounter, even with a sponsor.)

The emphasis on competition raises an important issue. In comparing various models of such care around the world, the competitive strategy is very American and, perhaps, appropriate to the entrepreneurial values of this society. However, the competition does come at a cost. In the alternative model, there would be an assignment of geopolitical responsibility through a public body or its designee. This body would be responsible for providing the necessary care to the designated population in a public utility mode. The advantages of the latter approach are simplification and easier accountability. Because everyone in the service area is covered under the single agency's umbrella, the need for risk rating is greatly reduced. Despite Professor Enthoven's plaudits for AAPCC in Medicare, that system has not been well received and does appear to present real problems. A much more sophisticated system will be needed to assure that there is not discrimination against the higher-risk clients, especially among the elderly. In a universal system, the elderly are likely to be especially discriminated against. If one is going on to propose, as Professor Enthoven has, experiments akin to the SHMOs, the chances of discrimination and the need for better predictors of risk are paramount concerns in a competitive strategy, even a managed competition. He does not address the question of what happens to those not enrolled. In the less-regulated new world of medical competition, we have grown accustomed to the talk about market niches and tend to forget that they produce market chinks, which are usually left as the residual responsibility of the public sector (too often with the ironic accusation that such care is then less efficiently delivered than that provided privately).

At the same time, there is indeed virtue in the spirit of competition. Professor Enthoven's proposal attempts to garner the best of both worlds. Beyond the general belief that competition promotes a better product, managed competition provides better data about the success of a plan's performance by monitoring the disenrollments and hence giving more credibility to consumer reaction. It provides alternative sources of care, which permits closing down a plan that does not perform satisfactorily. The problems of successfully regulating monopoly utilities are notorious.

We are caught then on the horns of an important dilemma—one which deserves careful debate. The competitive approach implies a great deal more work in identifying risks and paying appropriate premiums that will fairly attract enrollment in all sectors. Its monitoring activities will be more complicated by a similar need to conduct careful case adjustments. To be truly effective, it must assure meaningful, universal access. The benevolent sponsor appears as some form of deus ex machina with no clear indication of just how he would provide such assurance. The noncompetitive-utility approach offers more assurance of universal coverage but presents problems of enforcing the regulations by offering no alternatives, or at least making it difficult to create any.

FINANCING

In the Competitive Medical Plan (CMP), the enrollees could come from the employed, the poor, or the elderly. The government (or more precisely, various governments) would make different levels of contributions to each group. The federal government would provide a subsidy equal to 40 percent of the premium cost of an efficient plan. States would then subsidize "a large part of the rest" for the poor. Medicare would presumably continue to pay for Part A coverage. Enthoven tentatively suggests that the federal subsidy for Part B would be done on a means-test basis, but also provides for universal Medicare coverage and payroll taxes if any gaps are left.

The argument for the 40 percent subsidy is based on the idea that the consumer should be given the incentive to choose an efficient health care plan. Presumably if the full cost were paid, this incentive would be lost. It is not immediately clear to me why one could not take the next step and propose a simpler system, wherein the full cost (based on the cost of an efficient plan) were paid by the government (a euphemism for paid by us, but paid on a progressive-tax basis). This step would appear to have several advantages. It would simplify the proposal by eliminating the several tiers. It would retain the incentive to choose an efficient plan by paying at only that level, and it could pay for only the basic service package. It would remove the states from direct financial involvement, but it would mean escaping all the welfare-associated problems of determining eligibility, creating notches, and dealing with those who fall through the cracks.

I commend Professor Enthoven for pointing out the fallacy of the rhetoric about the costs of universal coverage. In his analysis of the cost implications, Professor Enthoven suggests that there are large pockets of potential savings represented by the existing, unfair subsidies paid under the personal and corporate tax structure. At the risk of challenging a respected economist at his own game, I wonder if he has even under-estimated the situation. If one were to add the costs of health care built into the goods and services the government purchases, the figure would likely even better offset the apparent costs of a universal health insurance model.

QUALITY

Professor Enthoven has done an important service in emphasizing the importance of quality measures. However, I fear that he may be too optimistic about the inherent capacity of health plans to monitor their own quality. He argues that quality and economy usually go hand in hand, akin to the old saying that it is cheaper to do a job well. Alas, there are many areas of quality that do not necessarily save money in either the long or the short run. The large bulk of medical care consists of treatments for problems where the intervention may have little or no effect on morbidity, to say nothing of mortality. Unless one is prepared to measure outcomes of care in much broader parameters that address the psychological aspects, best may not be cheapest. Perhaps allowing his disaffection for fee-for-service care to persuade him of the advantages of prepaid practice, he argues that increasingly cohesive CMPs will have incentives to improve quality for the sake of their reputations and economy. Such care provides the opportunity, but not necessarily the incentive, to monitor quality.

In the same presentation, however, he does correctly note the importance of outcomes of care among groups of people. Many health care philosophers have argued for a shift in the nature of future competition from price to quality. As we move into an era of population-based practice, we need to refocus our concepts of quality control from individual events to group data. In essence, we are moving into an era of epidemiologically measured performance—one in which we compare batting averages rather than swings at the ball. The shift is thus one from assessing the process of care to concentration on the outcomes of care. An important component of the outcomes is consumer satisfaction, an element directly addressed in a competitive model.

Professor Enthoven has correctly noted that a critical dimension of quality control is the dissemination of good information to the consumers. This task is too large to be undertaken without both an adequate support system and a sufficient population under observation to permit meaningful rate calculations. In fact, there is reason here to argue for national standards to assure comparability across areas as well as within them and, hence, an important role for the federal government.

OUTCOMES OF CARE

I would like to see us consider an even closer link between the outcomes of care and payment. We have already noted that the managed-competition system will require careful attention to population characteristics to calculate risks and measure outcomes of care. Why not use this data to provide even stronger incentives to plans by paying more for appropriately adjusted better outcomes? Under the Enthoven system, outcomes become the criteria used to assure an acceptable level of performance. I propose that this concept be expanded to its logical conclusion. We ought to be willing to pay more for better care and less for worse care. In truth, we will not likely shut down, or even greatly change, enrollment for even modest changes in most performance measures. Professor Enthoven is likely correct that most of the current competition is focused around access. If we really do restrict the benefit packages, access will become even more important as a competitive feature. If we wish to encourage quality, defined here in terms of outcomes adjusted for case-mix, we should plan to take advantage of the full opportunity presented by the managed-competition system.

Indeed, the emphasis on outcomes will introduce an important discussion about just what we really mean by the outcomes of care. Up to now, we have assumed a generally shared understanding of that concept, but such an assumption is very likely misplaced. At the least, we likely do not yet have anything approaching consensus about how we value the various components of outcomes relative to each other. The discussions about these usually revolve around standard measures of mortality and morbidity, but we have not ascertained how different segments of the population feel about these. For example, how do we value risk reduction compared with prompt attention to minor symptoms with no functional benefit? What about access to treatment for rare catastrophic events compared with more common but less dangerous ones? How much is reassurance worth? We talk about the need for greater attention to prevention but are not clear about what we might be willing to pay for it or trade for it. Moreover, in accepting an outcome-driven definition of quality, we have developed a system in which both the provider and consumer play important determining roles, but only the provider seems to be at risk.

Professor Enthoven has acknowledged the problem inherent in any capitated system, namely the danger of risk aversion creating selective enrollment and selective disenrollment. The sponsor may serve to protect against the former, especially if the appropriate risk measures can be implemented to set a fair price, but the problems of the latter are substantial. In all prepaid care there is the obvious incentive toward underservice. Monitoring outcomes offers some protection against that in the long run. Monitoring disenrollments offers a mechanism to note the phenomenon, but something more tangible needs to be offered to assure the elderly that they will get the benefits promised and that their only alternative is not simply leaving—since that penalizes the victim more than the provider. The experience with Medicare HMOs in the Twin Cities suggests that this is a matter of some concern. Although there are no hard data to estimate the true extent of selective disenrollment, the testimony of both Senate committees provides enough anecdotal data to make this an area for close attention. Better risk pricing will help somewhat, and sponsor attention with the risk of defamed reputation might be a modest deterrent, but neither of these seems sufficient.

WHAT WILL WORK? INVESTOR-OWNED VERSUS NONPROFIT

In the end, it is difficult to imagine a system of care (or payment for care) that will work easily in the United States. The strong entrepreneurial tradition suggests that the providers will find a way around any set of incentives that we propose. Nonetheless, managed competition appears to be a valiant effort to move away from the entrenched fee-for-service approach in a manner consistent with current trends. Essentially I agree with Professor Enthoven's observation that the economic performances of investor-owned systems and the not-for-profits have not been very different, although the accusations of selective marketing and patient dumping seem to be more frequently directed toward the former. Indeed, a recent study suggests that even in the Veterans Administration hospitals there is an excess of surgery similar to that described for the private sector. I am less sanguine that the difference between the two approaches lies in the public policies they espouse. Both are going to act in their own perceived best interest. I do not see why the not-for-profits will be more concerned with assuring widespread access to care. Both will be anxious to assure that there are comfortable markets for the kind of care they want to deliver. The institutions most concerned with access to care are the public ones. They are the sources of last resort and, hence, are the victims of market niching.

Nonetheless, I share Professor Enthoven's conclusion that it would be preferable to allow the values of the nonprofit sector to predominate. I believe that the concern with access will continue to be an important issue if we move into managed competition. The argument for nonprofit sponsorship is better couched in terms of public accountability. In an area where gaming is very likely to occur, I would rather have the players be accountable to board members who gain their prestige from their public image than to those interested primarily in enhancing the bottom line.

LONG-TERM CARE

An area of great concern to any discussion about health care for the elderly must be long-term care. There is growing recognition, even in some quarters of the government, that this represents the real catastrophic care. I was thus very pleased to note that Professor Enthoven dismissed the futile efforts to address this important issue with some form of private insurance. His analysis of the illogic of such an approach is commendable. I strongly endorse his position that we need a universal, mandatory social insurance program to cover long-term institutional care, but I question the narrowness of the target. I suspect his caution is based on a concern about defining such care too broadly, but it is misplaced. Surely long-term care is one area where the site of care is not the appropriate means to define the service. Having taken medicine to task for the chaos created by perverse incentives, he surely would not want to see the same inappropriate emphasis on institutional care in long-term care.

An approach very similar to the managed-care model seems well suited to long-term care. An issue of great concern is where the power should lie. Professor Enthoven recommends HMOs as indispensible bases for the development of SHMOs, his best candidate for solving the problem of integrating services to support the care of the frail elderly in noninstitutional settings. Leaving aside the apparent discrepancy with respect to care setting, the critical question is how to effectively merge social and medical care. Certainly more experimentation is needed, but what sort of experiments? The SHMO model allows for considerable latitude in how the two components are organizationally linked. Most elderly do not need long-term care at any time, and probably less than half will ever need it; but virtually all elderly persons will need health care. How then do we merge these two operations? Pooling resources leads us back into long-term care insurance, the very route disparaged.

The Canadian example suggests that the better answer may lie in not trying to marry the two forms of care too closely to the point of service.

Once universal coverage for health care has been assured, similar universal coverage of long-term care can be assured under separate but equal auspices. However, the latter is better developed from a social base than from a medical one. The long-term care system can be similarly capitated based on a risk model, with measures of accountability resembling those proposed for the CMP. The availability of social services should in no way affect the access to medical care, although the need for long-term care will inevitably affect the risk rating of the client. There is the potential for cost shifting at higher levels by reassigning resources from one sector to another in a manner similar to other decisions made about general resource allocations. The specific arrangements for coordination between the medical and social service systems will probably be best worked out at the local level.

The argument for a single source of medical and long-term care revolves around the potential efficiencies to be gained from such an arrangement. It may indeed prove feasible to work out a cooperative system for pooling resources. Opportunities of this sort should be encouraged, but it is important to recognize that when medical and social services are closely linked, the former usually dominate. Indeed, a careful examination of the SHMO programs as practiced suggests that they offer much less long-term care than the concept implies. Medical and social agencies may be able to work together, but they will probably do so best under conditions that allow the social agency to purchase services from the medical providers.

A BASE ON WHICH TO BUILD

In summary, Professor Enthoven has proposed an innovative approach for achieving some level of universal health insurance. He has built from a belief that our society will not abandon the job-related health care financing. His proposal is thus a compromise. He offers a sponsor who will continually oversee and adjust the American spirit of competition to assure that it responds to needs of clients. He seems to favor a public entity for this sponsor role, or at least a nonprofit agency. Within this controlled environment, he sees competition as the means to promote the best—most efficient—care, but he advocates careful accountability in terms of outcome measures and fair competition in terms of quality and access rather than price. There are still some gaps in his system. For example it is not totally clear why he doesn't drop the other shoe and move all the way to a simpler government-financed system with different sources of contribution. He has not yet truly tackled the question of how to integrate long-term care into a medical system. He has recognized some of the problems inherent in his proposal and has offered some basic, but likely inadequate, remedies. Nonetheless, it represents a promising base on which to build. It is an intriguing beginning, which may appeal to conservative elements as well as some liberals. (The former may see it as a ceiling and the latter as a floor.)

4

THE U.S. HEALTH CARE SYSTEM: BASIC GOALS

Robert L. Kane

The goals for a health care system are generally discussed under the headings of access, quality, and cost. This is true for the health care system of the United States as well. What has changed is the order of priority. Whereas the focus in the 1960s—the era of Medicare and Medicaid—was on access and quality, attention today has shifted to cost. The other concerns remain, however. It should be possible to provide care for all Americans (i.e., residents of this country) that is of an acceptable quality without reducing them to penury. If some form of rationing or limitations of benefits is required, such decisions should be debated in a context where everyone has a common stake.

My goal for a health care system in the United States is one based on universal coverage that includes a broad range of benefits for both acute and long-term care. The specific implementation of this approach might vary within defined parameters from location to location. A key principle of such a system, especially in a country so large and heterogeneous as the United States, is local control. With control, however, comes responsibility and accountability.

This need for feedback means that the operating system must have some method of working under constrained resources. For most purposes this means some form of capitated payment, though in this instance some method of accurate risk adjustment will be essential to avoid gross unfairness or manipulation. In the system evisioned, it is not necessary that both acute and long-term care services be operated by the same agency, though there are some advantages to such an arrangement, such as facilitating trade-offs and investments in different modes of care designed to avoid future loss. A cogent argument can be made that long-term care is primarily a social service, but it will always rely on effective links to acute medical care from physicians and hospitals. Such care can be purchased separately if there is too great a fear that the medical forces will overwhelm the social nature of the basic care.

I have publicly extolled the virtues of the Canadian system, especially as it merges long-term with acute-care coverage (Kane and Kane, *A Will and a Way*, 1985). The fundamental principle of universal coverage has been well implemented in Canada. Although the precise nature and extent of benefits vary from province to province, the general principles of coverage are mandated by federal law. In several provinces the acute and long-term care programs operate separately. Although they may be responsible to the same ministry and, hence, are funded from a common pool, they are administered independently. Under this arrangement, once major allocation decisions between acute and long-term care have been made centrally, the programs pursue their independent goals with whatever degree of coordination can be negotiated or mandated. Each pool is protected from raids by the other, but at the cost of some potential losses in efficiency.

Americans love to beat the game. Whatever the rules, we will try to get around them. Thus, the best rules are those that allow the player a chance to win by doing what is good for the system. In the case of health care, this means rewarding quality based on outcomes and spreading the risk as far as possible.

At the same time, I do not believe it is feasible nor appropriate to attempt to adopt wholesale the system of another country. Part of the tax on importing ideas from abroad is the appreciation that the values of each land are different, and values play a critical role in shaping social services such as health care.

The American solution will have to be uniquely American. It must recognize the entrepreneurial spirit that is endemic to this country. Americans love to beat the game. Whatever the rules, we will try to get around them. Thus, the best rules are those that allow the player a chance to win by doing what is good for the system. In the case of health care, this means rewarding quality based on outcomes and spreading the risk as far as possible. Concentrating the payment in a single entity allows the game to be focused rather than having the players compete for the best terms of market niches. I therefore favor a governmentally run system, though some form of intermediary may be used to administer the system, and the actual care should be given by private contractors held accountable by independent overseers hired by the government. Given the diversity of geography, ethnicity, and styles of practice, I would opt for some form of capitation that would equalize the investment after controlling for risk but would leave sufficient room for variations in approach. I am still uncertain about the trade-offs between competition among firms for markets and the advantage of geopolitical accountability.

A comprehensive system of universal coverage for acute and long-term care will make more overt the costs of care but need not increase the aggregate costs, except to the extent that those now prevented from getting care because of inability to pay may become users. At the same time there is a real possibility that centralizing (not necessarily into a single location, but even on a geographical basis) the sources of payment will readily provide opportunities for cost control that are not available under the current fragmented arrangements. Competition and cost control can coexist.

Although I prefer a truly universal system that includes everyone, I am willing to compromise on several points. First, we have the opportunity to begin with at least a segment of the population; namely, the elderly and the other groups covered under Medicare. Although a biased sample, these groups are now covered by a form of universal insurance that is not comprehensive. One feasible direction to make a beginning is to expand the coverage for these persons to include long-term as well as acute care and to broaden the acute coverage to include some obvious omissions such as ambulatory drugs. I dislike this strategy for philosophic and political reasons, primarily because it focuses attention on the elderly exclusively at a time when there is great concern about intergenerational equity.

Because we have maintained the myth that private and public dollars are subject to different principles of accounting, expanding the publicly funded benefits for a segment of the population will appear as a shift in total resources spent on the elderly. At a minimum, the financing of such a move must not appear to show a transfer of funds. Better information about the real costs of care must be made available. Public education is required to counteract the prevalent philosophy that good administration means transferring the problem to someone else's jurisdiction. The place to begin is with a clearer explication of the underlying dilemma—the need to spread risks widely and to control costs through an efficient and equitable means of rationing. In such a process, universal coverage implies a strong role for government. Shifting the financing approach from a private tax subsidy to an overtly public system that relies on insurance premiums of taxes does not change the nature of the funds collected.

A second level of compromise is to permit a variety of financing strategies. Under this approach, one might mandate that everyone be covered to at least a minimally designated extent but allow greater latitude in how that coverage is achieved. Thus, employer-based coverage might continue or even be mandated for a broader range of workers, leaving the unemployed to be covered by more directly public means. Again, this strategy is more appearance than substance. Its success depends in part on the ability to require that all the insurance purchased be administered in a similar fashion regardless of purchaser.

Because the employer payments are likely to continue to be tax deductible, the true fiscal difference between an overtly universal program and this sort of multisponsored approach is less than might first appear, but it has the advantage of appearing to be more consistent with a spirit of free enterprise. The danger lies in the growing interest of corporations to take a more active role in controlling health care costs. Once they get into this pattern, they will not be willing to simply pay into a pool over which they have little or no control. Many corporations have established active programs of managed care designed to reduce health care costs. Perhaps the best known example is that operated by Chrysler (Califano 1986). Although it is not clear how well these approaches have worked, many of the corporations employing them seem to value them very highly and would not likely give up such efforts if they were still required to contribute directly to health insurance benefits.

The argument that an active private market is the best way to assure quality and to set a standard does not offset the concern that such an independent market threatens to siphon off resources and makes it much harder in fact to ration care on an equitable basis. The more fragmented the market, the greater the opportunity for providers to play one group of consumers off against the others.

FINANCING THE SYSTEM

In the end, the simplest solution seems like the best. Why not use a universal coverage funded from a universal payment? In the simplest case, this boils down to either funding the system from taxes or using some means of mandating fees paid into the program, such as in a compulsory health insurance program. My own preference is for a tax-based system. It will be easier to administer and more conducive to a progressive rate structure. However, the insurance approach, akin to the Social Security Trust, offers greater protection from political action.

The distinction between a tax-based financing system and some form of compulsory health insurance lies essentially in the way the payment is determined. The goals of insurance, however, are to spread risk. We began health insurance with a strong commitment to community rating and proceeded to get into trouble by moving to various techniques to market policies on the basis of risk. In fact, it was risk-based rating that led to Medicare, because the elderly were priced out of the health insurance market when insurance companies began competing for the market presented in fringe-benefit packages by offering lower rates to working-age people. The risk was no longer spread, and health insurance rates for the elderly were unaffordable. If we go back to some form of community rating—at least for purposes of generating income—then the distinctions between compulsory insurance and taxes diminish. The former provides targeted funds that presumably are kept in a special account separate from general revenues and sheltered from the political process. The distinction between an insurance mechanism and taxation is often confused with public and private payment. Indeed, it is possible to have compulsory private funding.

Any effort to carry to the public the debate over private versus public funding of health care will require a better explication of how care is currently financed. Much of the public contribution is presently obscured. Tax subsidies, both to corporations and individuals, are not easily visible to the average person and are often undercounted even by the interested economist. Consider forgiveness of bad debts to hospitals, shifted burdens for uncovered care to private insurance that are then passed on as tax deductions, the cost of health insurance built into the costs of goods and services purchased by all levels of government from the private sector, and the governments' own costs of health insurance. These items consistently do not show up in calculations of contemporary public subsidies for health care over and above the obvious payments for public insurance (e.g., Medicare and Medicaid) and direct provision of care by publicly run facilities.

In the case of long-term care, for example, a substantial proportion of the funds labeled out-of-pocket are in fact transferred from Social Security payments and, to a lesser degree, from SSI. These go toward the cost of nursing home care but are counted as private payments because they go first to the beneficiary; still, they are mandatorily given to the nursing home. In fact, they explain some of the discrepancy between the amount of nursing home care paid by Medicaid and the number of people in nursing homes supported by Medicaid. We often hear figures that indicate Medicaid pays for almost half of the nursing home care in this country, but about two-thirds of the nursing home residents are supported in whole or in part by Medicaid.

Another argument for public funding through a more centrally operated mechanism like taxation is the ability to make distributional decisions at a sufficiently high level that the individual case is not confused with the policy involved. The first task of a system is to allocate resources in large blocks. Difficult choices must be made between health and education, between transportation and welfare. Health funding should be part of that process. Policies that go the next step, emphasizing one form of care over another (e.g., acute versus long-term, hospital versus ambulatory) are probably more easily made at a level removed from the direct pressures of individual clients and providers.

Rationing can occur in two ways. One can discourage access to services as is done in the United Kingdom, with expensive therapies such as renal dialysis for the elderly, or in the United States, where certain costs also provide a major barrier. Alternatively, one can limit the amount of service available to an individual on the basis of assessed need or even ability to pay. Presumably, once that amount of care is used, the client is no longer eligible. Obviously, in some circumstances, such a rule may be hard to enforce once the services have begun. Although we want to maintain flexibility to respond to individual client needs, rationing decisions or some form of discretionary limitations on resources are much more likely to be enforced at a level removed from direct contact with clients. As Aaron and Schwartz (1984) showed, rationing depends on consumers' and primary care providers' acceptance of the concept. Few providers can actually refuse care if it is demanded.

A program for financing comprehensive care for the elderly as a partial solution or preliminary step along the way to universal coverage should take special pains to avoid the appearance of further supporting the elderly on the backs of the workers. One step in this direction would be a full tax on Social Security payments, even at the risk of claims of double taxation. Another symbolically sound idea is increasing inheritance taxes. Perhaps other special tax benefits for the elderly might be used as well. The goal of the financing system should be to spread the burden among beneficiaries, not all taxpayers, in accordance with ability to pay. However, such a means test is better accomplished by taxation than by differential payments on use.

We must consider two steps in the discussion of strategies. Should universal health insurance be pursued directly or incrementally? If the latter, what happens to the rest of the system? Philosophically, I prefer to go for the whole pie rather than break it up, but there are compelling political arguments for a more indirect approach. The very numbers involved are frightening, and deliberate or careless use of them can be even more alarming if people perceive the costs somehow as new costs rather than the transfer of private dollars to public ones—simply collected by a different mechanism. Because Medicare represents an existing framework of universal coverage for a portion of the population with modest benefits to those eligible, it is tempting to begin there and build on that framework to add long-term coverage. The resultant model could then be used as a template to extend this coverage to the entire population.

CONTROLLING COST

The way a system is financed does not necessarily determine how it is organized. Universal coverage is compatible with fee-for-service payment (as exists in Canada) or a national health service like the United Kingdom's. It is similarly compatible with capitation, as is developing in this country. It is very likely that capitation will become an important part of health care organization in the United States. There are several compelling reasons. From the consumers' vantage point, it offers a limitation on cost and a simplification of what has become a very complex system of recovering expenses. Anyone who has struggled with the Medicare claim forms or has tried to understand the billing system will quickly appreciate why a prepaid system that requires no forms and sends no bills is very attractive, especially to older clients.

With the growth in direct out-of-pocket payments by beneficiaries, the idea of limiting risk and capping out-of-pocket costs is increasingly appealing to the public and to the government. The recent enthusiasm for catastrophic health care coverage speaks to the widespread concern about the costs of health care to individuals. One can protect individuals by limiting their liability or by developing other contracts to share the risk with providers through some form of prepaid care. From the government's perspective, capitation offers a mechanism to limit its financial commitment to a planable amount. Moreover, it removes the government from the politically turbulent area of rationing at the individual-client level. Painful decisions about limitations of service are made by groups distinct from the government. The decisions are no less painful; they are simply isolated.

It does not appear realistic to assume that we can avoid painful rationing decisions. Schwartz (1987) has argued that simply eliminating the so-called inappropriate care will not control our expenditures on health care. It will only move the curve back a little, leaving the slope untouched. The press of technology will continue to escalate costs. New health technologies often do not save money. They may be more effective, but even then it is at a price. Many have questioned the marginal benefits of these advances, but their appeal is well established. Americans have become technology junkies. We want the latest and assume that it is the best. In the current system, the providers of care are also the advocates for these new technologies. They share our fascination with novelty, while gaining prestige and income from the changes in practice style.

The only feasible way to control technology and, hence, health costs seems to be by relying on some form of capitation. Indeed, any major intervention by the government is in one sense a form of capitation in that it takes a set of revenues and must then provide services from the pool of resources. States forbidden to operate in a deficit are forced into some form of rationing. However, for our purposes, capitation implies some form of risk sharing by the providers of care. The most common forms are the HMO and the PPO. The rise of corporate practice of medicine seems very likely, if not inevitable, although the predictions of some about giant medical corporations akin to the oil conglomerates need not hold.

The question then is how will capitation work? One scenario calls for competition among different firms. This assumes that consumers will be able to distinguish between the quality offered and relate it to price. Presumably, different benefit packages will be available at different prices. Anyone who has struggled to buy more concrete goods, like tires, can imagine the difficulty that a consumer motivated to make an intelligent choice might face confronted by an array of claims and an assortment of facts. Good choices about health care are difficult to make by knowledge-able people, let alone the average consumer. Even providers appear to vary in their practice styles, with no clear empirical basis to justify the differences. Confidence in the free market suggests a belief that appears to exceed knowledge.

The inherent danger in a capitated system is the incentive for providers not to provide services or to provide as few as they can. The consumer has little real protection against this underservice. Although HMOs like to claim that consumers can vote with their feet by taking advantage of the open disenrollment clause, consumers who leave because they are not getting the service they deserve may be cheerfully dismissed. HMOs rely on the nonusers to balance their budgets. Losing a high-user client may be regarded with relief—due to losing a liability. Unless the consumer is prepared to go to court, simply relying on the marketplace does not seem to be enough.

The choice, then, within the capitated options lies with either a competitive system with strict controls enforced by some external agency (such as Enthoven proposes elsewhere in this volume) or a franchise approach that eliminates competition and thereby encourages responsibility. In such a system the provider cannot lose the consumer, but there needs to be some regulatory body that will enforce quality standards to avoid abuse and underservice. This is the equivalent of a utility model. The alternative is to impose on the competitive strategy some constraints. For example, we might require that any HMO from which a client withdraws will continue to be responsible for the costs of that client in the new HMO for a period, say a year.

If this concept is coupled with the other important aspect of capitation—namely, meaningful risk rating—the result would be a strong disincentive to encourage expensive clients to disenroll. Risk rating is an important part of capitation. We need better ways to estimate the impending care costs for different individuals if we want to avoid selective marketing. The goal of capitation is to encourage efficient care but not selection bias. Therefore, we want a pricing system that will set the risks fairly. Under such a system, a client who disenrolls from an HMO would be independently reevaluated, and a new risk rating would be calculated. However, the former HMO would be responsible for the difference in the price of the new rating compared with the old. In essence, it would continue to bear the financial risk (at the pooled level) for the next coverage period.

It is still too early to tell just how effective prepaid group practice will be as a national phenomenon. Although enrollments have grown substantially of late, most of the population is still using the fee-for-service approach. In a country as heterogeneous as the United States, no single approach will likely prevail. The corporate approach described above may evolve in several different forms that will combine different aspects of physician choice and payment mechanisms. All will have in common an overall accountability and responsibility for the amount and quality of care.

ASSURING QUALITY

Capitation provides a special opportunity to assure quality. We have already made some significant strides with regard to our technology for quality assessment. We have moved beyond structure to look at the process of care. We were appropriately less interested in a person's qualifications than in what that person did. We have moved even further now to focus on the outcomes of care. The operation can no longer be considered a success if the patient dies. We are beginning to see a burgeoning of sophisticated data systems designed to measure the outcomes of care. So far the definitions of outcomes have been pretty narrow. We tend to begin and end with the hospital, though the results of hospital care may not be truly evident for some time after discharge. We are nonetheless beginning to think in terms of health care careers, in which the client's experience is viewed as a continuum. Certainly, the links between acute and long-term care require just such a perspective (Lewis et al. 1985; Kane and Matthias 1984).

People do not stop being long-term care clients when they enter a hospital or visit a physician, nor do they begin such careers at a sharply differentiated point on leaving the hospital. The very nature of geriatric practice is predicated on the concept of investment. The operant belief calls for a willingness to provide intensive evaluation and treatment, with the expectation that this effort will result in improved functioning and, ultimately, in reduced cost. Data from a number of programs for geriatric assessment suggest that more careful attention to patients' long-term care needs during the acute phase of their illness can produce better treatment plans, which will in turn reduce the cost of subsequent long-term care (Rubenstein 1987). Conversely, better primary care to persons in long-term care situations can reduce subsequent use of expensive acute care, such as hospitals (Kane et al. 1976; Master et al. 1980).

If the payment systems for acute care are derived from separate sources than those from long-term care, as is the case with Medicare and Medicaid, there is little incentive to invest efforts in one sector with the expectation of recovering them in another. Medicare currently pays for hospital and physician services, but for very little nursing home care. Medicaid, virtually by default, becomes the major payor of nursing home care.

Within a sphere of care, outcomes can be successfully incorporated into the reward system. The present regulatory system relies on penalties (such as fines) levied for inadequate performance. There are problems with both defining the standards of care and enforcing the regulations; each confrontation becomes an invitation to litigation. If the ultimate sanction is closing a facility, the political pressure against doing so may be too great. A better approach to encouraging better care may lie in using outcomes as the basis of payment, or at least as a partial basis. Under such a strategy, the outcomes must be expressed in terms of expected outcomes in order to adjust for differences in case mix. The use of an outcome measure that is essentially a ratio of achieved outcome to expected outcome also avoids the problem of creaming, often associated with any payment system relying on levels of care. In a level-based system, the provider is always trying to choose the patient who is just over the next category, just as one might seek seats in the first row of the next cheapest section in a theater. Moreover, the incentive in a level-of-care system is perverse. The worse the patient becomes, the more the provider is paid. In an outcomes-based system the providers are encouraged to take the worst cases because almost any improvement or even delayed decline will show up as a course better than expected. The provider trying to game this approach would need a way to predict a patient's prognosis more accurately than the statistics driving the system. This is akin to the horse race bettor who has a system to beat the handicappers. The operant condition is clients achieving reasonable levels of performance, where the expectation is statistically determined from examples of good care. Achieving such good outcomes would trigger a bonus payment; achieving substantially suboptimal outcomes would generate a penalty. Such a system has been developed and piloted for nursing home care (Kane et al. 1983).

An important byproduct of such an approach is its flexibility. By focusing attention on the outcomes rather than on the process of care and by adjusting for differences in client characteristics, you are free to compare different modalities of care. Thus, the relative effectiveness of institutional versus community-based care can be tested and rewarded. Moreover, this sort of approach is compatible with various payment systems. It can be used to generate bonus payments in a capitated system or to adjust fees in a fee-for-service system.

However, an outcomes approach alters the responsibility for the outcome. It becomes a joint responsibility. Unlike the traditional measures, by which each step can be assessed individually, the price of permitting flexibility and creativity is the need to hold the whole production unit accountable as a unit. Although internal management procedures may monitor the subcomponents of care, the external responsibility is singular. Thus, an outcomes approach requires some form of corporate entity to take overall responsibility and to oversee the components.

The introduction of capitation raises a new set of opportunities to take the next major step in assuring quality. Up to now, we have been concerned about how to address the outcomes of services provided. The stimulus has been the receipt of services. At the same time, I have asserted that the pressing policy question of today and tomorrow is rationing—the failure to provide services. Capitation addresses that issue by looking at the parent population of enrolled persons. This epidemiological approach to quality asks this fundamental question: How is the health of the group affected by the care system? This question involves those who do not get care as well as those who do. It raises a number of important but perplexing issues. It demands that we look at how we value one set of outcomes relative to another. If we are to make any overall assessment about the health status of a group, we must first define the relevant domains and then determine their relative importance. Indeed, the importance may vary with the nature of the group under study. We may decide that prevention (or reducing risk) is less important for some people than for others. Nonetheless, we will have begun an important discussion that has not been often held about just what we really want or expect from the health care system. This transition to epidemiologic quality assessment is the next big step in the development of the field. It will come with the widespread introduction of capitation.

DECISION MAKERS

If the capitated scenario is indeed valid, the decision making occurs at several levels. I have already noted the fallacy of blindly assuming that free market principles will apply to health care. At a central level, within the corporation or the geopolitical unit of a franchise, major decisions about the size of relative investments in different sectors of care must be made. The allocation of resources, usually expressed in terms of money, is a prime determinant of the extent of activities in a sphere. In the Canadian situation, for example, within the provincial ministries of health, allocations among acute and long-term care are made, along with allocations to transportation and education. At the next level down, hospital expenditures are budgeted in terms of global budgets, based on past performance and planning. Similar allocations are made for community-based care by means of budgets for geographically designated areas.

Managers within each unit have general control of how the allocated resources are spent, with the usual demands of accountability based on demand and performance. Under a program of global budgeting, as with capitation, there are immediate incentives not to provide services. For example, Canadian hospitals complain about the long-stay patients as bed-blockers, but astute observers point out that these complaints may not be valid because with such cases, hospitals may maintain beds at a lower daily cost than if new patients were admitted. In a similar manner, in HMOs there is a strong incentive to substitute less expensive care for high-priced technology. Preventive services may thus be highly valued, not so much for their health benefits as for their low unit cost and attractiveness to a group of potential enrollees who are basically healthy. Thus, there emerges a tension between providers and consumers. The power of the consumer exists at the time of choosing to enroll rather than at the time of disenrollment. A strong and effective consumer presence will require a well-developed information base that contains information on the quality of services, the outcomes achieved across a wide spectrum of problems, the ease of access, and the extent of personal attention provided. Such information is not likely to be easily available from the providers. If the consumers are truly to use the power of the marketplace, they will need independent data. Government regulatory agencies may be the best source for such information.

In our society, the government has a role beyond that of a payor of care. We look to government agencies to assure the general quality of care through a system of licensure. Thus, the government's role will include several functions. As we move toward universal care, the government becomes a payor and, as such, has a direct stake in the quality of the services it purchases. To the extent that some form of franchising is used, there is an even stronger need to measure quality against some sort of fixed standards because comparisons may be harder to find. As a payor, the government has an exciting opportunity to link two important concepts that could avoid some of the current problems with regulation; namely, cost and quality. If payments contained some system for rewarding or penalizing for good or bad outcomes, respectively, there would be a direct-incentive system that should send clear market signals.

Applying an outcome-based system to an entire health care system means addressing a number of issues our society has carefully avoided. We will need some measures of what aspects of health status we truly value. We can measure the health status of groups of people and compare the changes in the group under the auspices of one system of care with the changes under another. Still, to make valid comparisons we need to weight the outcome measures in a way that reflects the values we attribute to the various components. How much do we really want to reduce risks of future disease through preventive efforts compared with treating acute problems—many of which may be self-limiting? At the same time, how much is it worth to relieve the anxiety that the problem is not serious? Do we feel the same about treating acute illness in persons with chronic disease as in those with no other apparent illnesses? Do we value mental and social well-being as much as physical health, as implied in the WHO definition of health? Do we value more the relief of pain than the treatment of underlying disease? These are just a sample of the kinds of value-based questions that derive from a focus on the outcomes of care rather than the process.

We have established a rather extensive capacity to measure health status among a variety of different groups. It is feasible to monitor changes in that status at regular intervals and even to analyze the results by subgroups adjusted for prior disease state or other pertinent risk factors. We have a much less well-developed system for valuing these states. Work in this arena will be critical to the development of systemwide outcome-based approaches.

ACCESS AND SCOPE OF COVERAGE

The system envisioned should be universal in benefits and coverage. In the best-case example, all permanent residents of the country should be eligible. Because such a step seems a big one to discuss in the context of federal budget deficits, we must consider a fallback position. Coverage for three major elements can be achieved by more modest-appearing changes in the current programs affecting the elderly (and the other groups covered by Medicare), the employed (and their dependents), and the poor (especially those covered by Medicaid). Proposals have already been made to require mandatory coverage of workers and their families. Medicare represents a form of universalism for an age-defined group. Medicaid has a number of disadvantages in terms of both determining eligibility and providing perverse incentives to impoverishment. Nonetheless, combining these three major programs under a single set of common standards would provide a level of coverage that would shape the entire field of health care.

The expansion of Medicare to include long-term care would address the problems of fragmentation of services for the elderly now so flagrant in the gaps between Medicare and Medicaid. It would nonetheless leave the morass of eligibility issues that confuse both consumers and providers. Any efforts in this direction need to confront directly the merger of coverage for acute and long-term care. Common benefits might exacerbate concerns over duplicate coverage, however, enhancing the present perverse incentives for different units of government to use those programs to which they contribute the least. Using several programs at the outset has the advantage of not focusing all activity on the elderly. On the other hand, as already noted, the elderly represent a logical starting point to build a program of universal coverage because of the base offered by Medicare. However, politically there are already great concerns about a shift of resources away from other segments of society, especially the young.

Another important event that may shape the future of health insurance is the growing epidemic of AIDS. Not only is this a disaster of plague proportions with all the attributes of an epidemic to create social disaster, the disease attacks the working-age population in a pattern that has become increasingly hard to predict as the disease relies on heterosexual transmission. The concept of universal risk among working-age people for catastrophic consequences sets the stage for universal health insurance as has no other recent event. The perverse coincidence that AIDS mocks many of the stages of declining function among the elderly suggests that many of the same long-term care problems must be faced for this group as well.

It seems very likely that the pressures created by the AIDS epidemic, especially as it spreads actively to the heterosexual population of working adults as predicted, will catalyze interest in some form of national health insurance. Here would be a disease of catastrophic personal and financial consequences for which all are potentially at risk and for whom corporations may be potentially liable. A means to spread the financial risk as widely as possible seems very attractive. The major alternatives will be either a specific expansion of Medicare to cover AIDS, as was done with end-stage renal disease (ESRD), or a push for national health insurance. The severe, untoward, unpredicted fiscal effects of specific inclusion of ESRD may encourage many to choose the latter option.

MODEL SYSTEMS

The searchers for a model of care can do well to look carefully at the Canadian system for some useful lessons (Kane and Kane, A Will and a Way, 1985). Here is a government-financed system supported in most provinces by taxes but in some by compulsory insurance premiums. Care is provided by private providers working under negotiated arrangements. Benefits include both acute-medical and long-term care services. The services are provided by a variety of agencies and providers. The long-term care is generally administered as social services, though it may be the responsibility of a health ministry. The programs are not the responsibility of social welfare programs. In fact, income support and health services are now quite separate. With the availability of universal coverage, income and health care are no longer related. Welfare programs like Medicaid are irrelevant; poverty is not a precondition to care. Important to thinking in the United States, all this has been accomplished at a lower level of total spending for health care compared with America. In fact, the proportion of GNP going to health care in Canada has been less than the United States since 1970. (Kane and Kane, *Feasibility*, 1985).

The Canadian system does not readily translate into American idiom. Ours is a more entrepreneurial society, in which regulation and incentives will dominate negotiation and accommodation. Thus, I have turned to approaches like capitation with great enthusiasm (and considerable caution) as a means of capping costs and limiting growth.

The ideal model integrates acute and long-term care, but even the Canadian example does not carry that off except at the level of provincial governments. It is indeed possible to address acute and long-term care separately, even to the point of capitating each independently. The experience with Medicare HMOs under the Tax Equity and Fiscal Responsibility Act of 1982 (TEFRA) suggests that such care is attractive to a number of older persons. The efforts to extend this concept to include even limited long-term care benefits through programs like the SHMO are just getting underway as very limited experiments. The strongest arguments for integration are based in the concept of recouping efforts in one sector for the other. If both areas are supported by the same payors—even if separately organized—that incentive persists, though it may operate at a more subtle level.

RECOMMENDATIONS

It is high time we had a program of universal health insurance in this country. The issue then is not whether we should have it, but what form it should take and how it can be introduced in the most politically acceptable way. In terms of the goals component, I recommend a comprehensive approach, which includes both acute and long-term care. I also believe that beyond the principles of coverage and general benefits, we will have to allow great leeway in a country as heterogeneous as ours. The structure of such a program will likely vary from place to place. It is not at all clear how tightly the major components must be bound together once there is a basic mechanism to prevent the isolation that now plagues the separation of Medicare and Medicaid. There are lots of models available to examine. Some combine acute and long-term care under a single system; most do not, feeling that one is more medical and the other more social. However, the central funding allows a shifting of resources to develop long-term care services, often with medical dollars.

On the question of political strategy, I must confess that I waffle. I basically prefer a direct approach that would combine all the programs under a single body in a region, preferably a governmental entity. That agency would then be empowered to contract for services in various forms. The program would be truly universal and, hence, would have the buying power of a monopsony and the potential to reshape the delivery system. However, the American public has been frightened by the specter of national health insurance and its price tag for so long that going straight for the goal may mean losing in a good cause. I would then prefer to win a series of smaller victories.

The debate over catastrophic health insurance has surfaced the importance of extending Medicare coverage to include long-term care. There seems to be pretty good support among much of the citizenry for maintaining and improving Medicare, whatever their feelings about the tendency to overserve the affluent elderly. It may therefore be more realistic to pursue an incremental approach, focusing first on expanding Medicare benefits and then using this expanded system as a template for universal coverage. This more gradual approach has another advantage. Each discussion of the strategies points out vividly how much we need to experiment and learn about alternative ways to mount and oversee services. Given the size and complexity of this country, we may simply not be ready to go forward whole hog. Using the Medicare experience as a learning and testing ground may be prudent. We do know that every time we develop a program, we create a new set of providers who become active political forces in shaping the next steps.

We should recognize the inherent advantages of a universal system of care that includes both acute and long-term care services. Given the size and complexity of the United States, any federal system will require active decentralization. Every Western nation with a program of national health insurance has relied on local governments to carry it out, including the Canadian experience, which is built around separate provincial health care systems operating under a broad set of national guidelines. We should note, too, that the average Canadian province has the population of our major cities or counties.

This is not a time for timidity. We need to educate the legislators and the public about the real costs of care and the burden already borne by public funds. We need a debate on what kinds of care we want and for whom. The emergence of AIDS as a major health problem will likely change the nature of this debate. The catastrophic threat to a large sector of working-age people may catalyze activities toward some form of national health insurance.

A universal program is better than one limited to already partially covered groups like the elderly; but the Medicare program needs to be expanded to include long-term care, either as part of a universal program or as a more targeted effort. Broadened coverage does not necessitate merged administration. Long-term care is still better approached as a social program in need of medical support. Although capitation seems likely to become the predominant mode of funding, a forced marriage of acute and long-term care should be avoided. Common funding and the elimination of current disincentives attributable to different sponsors and different regulations may be a sufficient and appropriate beginning for this merger.

More attention should be focused on measures of quality and ways to incorporate quality into provider incentives. Ideally we want to reward good care, especially good outcomes. More and better discussions of what we truly value from health care will be an essential and worthwhile byproduct of such activity. As we move toward capitation, we will need to address ways of measuring and rewarding health status for groups of persons. Again, we must examine more closely what we really want and what it is worth. Death and disease may not be the only measures to consider. Risk reduction and reassurance are also important components of care. With a better fix on outcomes of care, we can afford to be more creative in seeking new ways to deliver care.

REFERENCES

Aaron, H. J., and W. B. Schwartz. *The Painful Prescription: Rationing Hospital Care.* Washington, D. C.: The Brookings Institution, 1984.

Califano, J. *America's Health Care Revolution: Who Lives Who Dies Who Pays.* New York: Random House, 1986.

Kane, R. A., and R. L. Kane. "The Feasibility of Universal Long-Term Care Benefits: Ideas from Canada." *New England Journal of Medicine* 312: 1357–63 (1985).

Kane, R. L., L. A. Jorgensen, B. Teteberg, and J. Kuwahara. "Is Good Nursing Home Care Feasible?" *Journal of the American Medical Association* 235: 516–19 (1976).

———, and R. A. Kane. *A Will and a Way: What Americans Can Learn about Long-Term Care from Canada.* New York: Columbia University Press, 1985.

———, and R. Matthias. "From Hospital to Nursing Home: The Long-Term Care Connection." *Gerontologist* 24: 604–9 (1984).

———, R. Bell, S. Riegler, A. Wilson, and E. Keeler. "Predicting the Outcomes of Nursing-Home Patients." *Gerontologist* 23: 200–6 (1983).

Lewis, M. A., S. Cretin, and R. L. Kane. "The Natural History of Nursing Home Patients." *Gerontologist* 25: 382–88 (1985).

Master, R. J., M. Feltin, J. Jainchill, R. Mark, W. N. Kavesh, M. T. Rabkin, B. Turner, and S. Lennox. "A Continuum of Care for the Inner City: Assessments of Its Benefits for Boston's Elderly and High-Risk Populations." *New England Journal of Medicine* 302: 1434–40 (1980).

Rubenstein, L. Z. "Geriatric Assessment: An Overview of its Impacts." *Clinics in Geriatric Medicine* 3(1): 1–16 (1987).

Schwartz, W. B. "The Inevitable Failure of Current Cost-Containment Strategies: Why They Can Provide Only Temporary Relief." *Journal of the American Medical Association* 257: 220–24 (1987).

5

A CRITIQUE OF THE KANE PROPOSAL FOR THE U.S. HEALTH CARE SYSTEM

Karen Davis

The Kane view of the U.S. health care system is most developed as it relates to long-term care for the elderly. An understanding of the complete system can only be guessed by reading between the lines. At the considerable risk of putting ideas on paper that do not accurately reflect those of Kane, the following elements of a Kane-proposed system for health and long-term care in the United States are postulated:

- *Universal acute-care health insurance coverage*
  A key element of the Kane proposal is a universal system of coverage for acute health care. Given the pragmatic orientation of the Kane plan, it is assumed that this would be a mixed public–private system with financing from a combination of taxes and private health insurance premiums.
- *Universal long-term care coverage with comprehensive continuum of benefits*
  The Kane proposal would provide for universal long-term care coverage with financing largely through the public sector. Medicare might be expanded to cover long-term care, with a residual Medicaid program retained for those not covered by Medicare.
- *Decentralization of responsibility and authority*
  The Kane plan would devolve responsibility to manageable geopolitical units such as cities or counties. Federal funding would be allocated to local jurisdictions on a capitation basis. Ideally this capitation rate would include payment for acute and long-term care. Local authorities would be given considerable discretion to use such funds flexibly to meet the continuum of acute and long-term care needs of the population

within their jurisdiction. Federal guidelines and standards would set certain minimums that would be universally applicable.

- *Mixed public–private delivery system*
  Acute and long-term care services would be provided by a mix of public, nonprofit, and proprietary organizations.

- *Provider payment*
  Emphasis would be placed on capitation payment of providers, with rewards for good health outcomes or high patient satisfaction. These rewards would be based on deviations from predictions of outcomes to avoid rewarding those who selected the easiest or healthiest patients. While provider organizations would be paid on a capitation basis, individual providers within the organizations may be paid on a fee-for-service or contractual basis. For example, health maintenance organizations would be paid capitation rates, and individual hospitals or physicians would be paid on a contractual or fee-for-service rate by the HMO. The DRG prospective payment system for hospitals would be eliminated.

- *Family role*
  Families would be encouraged to provide support to patients requiring long-term care. Day care and respite care would be available to provide necessary relief for families, particularly those caring for seriously dependent patients such as Alzheimer's patients. Support groups or therapy and counseling for caregivers would also be available.

- *Entry into long-term care services*
  Long-term care services would be coordinated by a gatekeeper or care coordinator. Patients would be assessed to determine their need for services. Emphasis would be placed on care in the community. Services would include nursing home care (but this would be used only when no other alternative was feasible), home nursing services, and homemaking services. Patients in nursing homes would pay the "housing cost" of such care. Hours of homemaking services per month would be based on the assessment of patient need. Home nursing and homemaking services would be either provided by salaried public employees or purchased from for-profit or nonprofit agencies. A wider variety of housing arrangements would be encouraged, including sheltered housing and lifecare communities.

- *Quality*
  Considerable emphasis would be given in the Kane system to the measurement and monitoring of quality of care provided. Specific economic rewards for good quality would be built into the payment system. Quality would be measured largely by patient outcomes, rather

than by process indicators. These outcome measures would encompass physical, cognitive, social, and emotional functioning as well as patient satisfaction. The Kane plan would upgrade the workforce providing long-term care services through better pay and investment in the selection, orientation, and ongoing training of such workers.

CRITIQUE OF THE KANE PLAN

Acute Care

The Kane plan is very sketchy as it applies to acute health care coverage in the United States. The role of employer health insurance plans is not clear. No explicit plan is presented for covering the 35 million Americans without any health insurance coverage. Reform of the acute-care portion of Medicare (e.g., placing a ceiling on out-of-pocket expenses of the elderly, merging Part A and Part B, improving drug coverage) is not discussed. Nor is there any suggestion of how such improvements in acute-care coverage for different population groups might be financed. Kane does note that transferring expenditures from the private sector to the public sector should not be viewed as new costs and seems generally sympathetic to greater public financing of acute health care expenditures.

The one intriguing reference to acute care is the possibility of diverting funds from acute care to long-term care. While this reference is not spelled out in any detail, it appears to refer to incentives for reducing hospitalization in a system of capitation payment for organizations providing both acute and long-term care. For example, lifecare communities may succeed in reducing hospitalization rates by providing a more supportive living environment with ready access to nursing and social services. If lifecare communities were to receive a capitation rate for acute-care benefits based on the risk of patients living in such communities, savings from reduced hospitalization could be used to subsidize long-term care services.

The proposal to try a wider variety of capitation payment systems seems worthy of further exploration. Even short of a major reform, demonstration of a variety of capitation payment systems for entities providing both acute and long-term care should be tried—well beyond the quite limited Social Health Maintenance Organization demonstration currently underway. As corporate entities are being established that encompass a network of providers such as hospitals, nursing homes, home health agencies, senior citizen housing, etc., greater opportunities for experimentation with this approach are created. Legislation to overcome the division between Medicare financing of acute care and Medicaid financing of long-term care may be necessary to facilitate such payment demonstrations.

Long-Term Care

The most innovative portion of the Kane plan pertains to long-term care. Considerable thought has been given primarily to how the delivery system might be made more responsive to individual patient needs and preferences. Again, the Kane plan favors some form of universal long-term care financing, though the specific details are not provided. The Canadian approach of a block capitation grant from the federal government to local government seems preferred, with local governments adding funds necessary to assure the availability of a continuum of long-term care services.

The Kane plan seems primarily useful in pinpointing interesting areas for further demonstration and kinds of provisions that should be built into any long-term care system developed for the United States, such as the gatekeeping-assessment function, support for caregiving families, and greater attention to mechanisms for upgrading and assuring quality of care.

The portions of the Kane plan that seem most feasible and that could be pursued independent of broader reform include:

- Broader coverage of respite services, including home-help care, day care, support groups, and counseling for caregivers of extremely dependent patients, such as those in advanced stages of Alzheimer's disease.
- Basing nursing home participation in Medicare and Medicaid on health outcome indicators and patient or family satisfaction. More attention to workforce orientation, training, and turnover should be part of the certification process rather than simple attention to numbers of nursing staff.

While the Kane plan provides several ideas conducive to more immediate application, in general I find the Kane plan too wide-sweeping to be politically or administratively feasible in the next ten years. The following aspects of Kane's plan are of particular concern:

- Transferring federal tax revenues to local jurisdictions to allocate. The history of block grant programs in the United States is that such programs are always underfunded because federal politicians are unwilling to take the political heat to raise taxes if the credit for the disbursement of funds goes to local politicians.
- Greater responsibility for local jurisdictions. The U.S. experience with Medicaid is quite different from the Canadian experience with national health insurance. The history of welfare medicine through state programs is one that would prove extremely difficult to shake in any new system vested in local government responsibility.
- Basing acute and long-term care payment on capitation. While capitation is an important long-term system of provider payment, the major methodological barrier is setting a rate that is appropriate given the health risk of the population covered. Extending capitation payment to the severely disabled population in need of long-term care only intensifies the problems of capitation payment and could lead to serious attempts to avoid enrolling those most in need of assistance. Considerable demonstration and experimentation will be required to solve this methodological problem.
- Health outcome measurement. Another feature of the Kane plan that seems a long way from practical implementation is the notion that provider payment could be based on whether health outcomes are better or worse than what would have been predicted. While the notion of including patient or family satisfaction with the quality of care in nursing home certification processes has great appeal, basing payment rates on a complex index of patient functioning seems far from ready for implementation. Some demonstration of this concept, however, would be worthwhile.

SUMMARY

In summary, the Kane plan needs considerable development before it could be translated into a specific legislative proposal. Definition of covered populations, benefit packages, cost sharing, if any, sources of financing, cost, administrative mechanisms, provider payment methods, etc., all need further elaboration. The general outline of the plan, however, is such a marked departure from the current U.S. health care system that I have serious doubts concerning its political and administrative feasibili-ty—even if such details were forthcoming. The Kane plan seems primarily useful in pinpointing interesting areas for further demonstration and kinds of provisions that should be built into any long-term care system developed for the United States, such as the gatekeeping-assessment function, support for caregiving families, and greater attention to mechan-isms for upgrading and assuring quality of care.

6

FINANCING HEALTH CARE: SOME BASIC CONSIDERATIONS

Robert G. Evans

The *Canada Health Act*, passed unanimously by the federal Parliament in April 1984, consolidates and clarifies prior federal legislation underlying the public, universal, comprehensive hospital and medical insurance systems in the provinces of Canada. In its preamble, it states that ". . . the primary objective of Canadian health care policy is to protect, promote and restore the physical and mental well-being of residents of Canada . . ."

This seems to me to be a reasonable summary of what Canadians expect their health care system to do. Certainly the legislation was overwhelmingly supported in national public opinion polls. I believe that some similar statement would command general assent in most other countries, including the United States.

HEALTH CARE, HEALTH, AND SOME SEMANTIC TRAPS

This statement of objectives, defined at least in principle in terms of health status or potentially measurable outcomes of care, distinguishes health care in a fundamental way from most of the other economic activities carried on in a community. Economists in particular commonly assume that the appropriate political or moral principle, the objective underlying those other activities, is or should be the very different concept of consumer sovereignty.

On this latter principle, it is postulated that the proper end of economic activity is to enable individuals to get what they want most, as judged by themselves. It is typically further assumed that the strength of their wants is best expressed by their willingness to pay, in turn reflected in their offers to do so, in a framework of voluntary exchange transactions. The sum total of such voluntary exchanges, the "free market," then determines what is produced, how, and for whom.

Consumer sovereignty, if applied to health care, implies that in this sphere as well, people ought to get what they are willing (and therefore by implication also able) to pay for, irrespective of any implications for their health. (Their willingness to pay may be based on their perceptions of health implications—but need not be—and in any case, such perceptions add no additional information to the transaction. The perceptions of observers other than the consumer are simply irrelevant.) This view is in stark contrast to the idea that the health care system is intended to promote the health of the community.

The two principles cannot be reconciled by analysis; neither can be shown to be in some objective sense "right" or "wrong," although they *do* have very different consequences in application. They are simply pre-analytic statements of values and beliefs. The assertion of the position that the health care system should serve to promote health, not to respond to individual offers to pay for particular goods and services, however, relies not only on my own values, but on the empirical observation that this is also the expressed view of the overwhelming majority of my fellow citizens. As noted above, I believe it is also the majority view, insofar as the matter has been thought out, in all other civilized countries—which I believe includes the United States.

If the proper function of the health care system is to promote health, then the health care *financing* system should be supportive of that objective. At the same time, however, since all resources are scarce, it should provide incentives for the efficient production of health. This implies efficiency in the conventional sense in the provision of health *care*. A good financing system should not encourage, or even leave undisturbed, unnecessarily costly patterns of production and waste of human time and talents. But it also, and most importantly, implies that the health care funding system must be concerned with *effectiveness*, with the relationship between care provided and health outcomes obtained. Ineffective care is waste, however efficiently it may be produced.

The concern for effectiveness most clearly distinguishes the values underlying health care provision from the principle of consumer sovereignty. Useless or care should not be provided or paid for, whether or not "consumers" can be found who are willing to pay for it. Nor should useful care be withheld from those who are "unwilling," which in practice almost always means simply unable, to pay for it. The standard of usefulness is effectiveness in achieving health outcomes, which are in principle identifiable by expert observers external to the care transaction.

Structuring health care systems so as to promote effectiveness remains a major policy challenge. But the arguments for professionalization and regulation in health care, both traditional and modern, have always rested on the assumption that an unregulated free market would lead to quackery, exploitation of the consumer, and adverse health outcomes. While there is no U.S. or international experience with a real free market in health care—no nation has ever wanted to take the risk—the evidence available so far from a number of countries indicates that the control of ineffective care within the context of a highly (self-) regulated industry is more feasible in a public, universal insurance system.

Adoption of the objective that the health care system should improve health outcomes or the health status of the community underlies the argument that the costs of providing health care should be distributed across the community in accordance with ability to pay rather than in accordance with utilization of services. The user-pay principle has very limited application in this area, being inconsistent with commonly held principles of equity as well as, in practice, with the promotion of efficiency.

The argument for the user-pay principle *appears* to have some basis in equity insofar as it implies contribution to health care finance in proportion to benefits received. But the concept of benefits received in health care rests on a semantic confusion. When health care is treated, conceptually and rhetorically, as a commodity, it becomes described in economic terms as a "good." By extension, users of health care are treated as having received benefits, associated with the use of these "goods," and it is easy then to infer that these "beneficiaries" ought to pay part, if not all, of the costs of such services.

Things look very different, however, when we view health care instrumentally, as a "regrettable" or necessary evil. If people value health care, not for itself, but because they believe they "need" it to remedy or prevent some illness, then the use of care marks the user off from nonusers not as more fortunate, a "beneficiary," but as *less* fortunate. (Note again the deceptive terminology borrowed from the insurance industry. *Beneficiaries* of insurance coverage are those who have *suffered* from some reimbursable event, such as accident, illness, or loss of home.)

To apply the "benefits received" principle in this context, by charging the user, adds economic loss to the noneconomic, but very real, costs of being ill—pain, fear, reduced ability to function—as well as to the economic costs that go beyond health care itself. If health care is a "good," it has a very close association with the "bads" of illness and injury.

Again, I think that the vast majority of my fellow citizens look at health care the same way, as a "regrettable," and that is why user charges are so often described in Canada as "taxing the sick." The appropriate thought experiment for the individual is to imagine oneself suffering any particular illness or health defect, yet being provided, free, with optimal care. Then consider not having the illness, or the care. Which state is preferred? The answer is easy in almost all cases; health is better.

Put another way, a person spending two weeks at a tropical resort is generally envied. A person spending two weeks in a hospital, using up a much larger allocation of "goods," is generally accorded sympathy, and with good reason. The user may be better off, *given that his or her health was threatened*, as a result of spending the time in the hospital. But the total impact of the episode, illness plus care, is unambiguously negative. This elementary fact is confused by the semantic trap of the economic language of "goods," and the neglect of the linkage between health care and health status.

UNIVERSAL AND COMPREHENSIVE COVERAGE: WHAT GROUNDS FOR DISCRIMINATION?

This rather long preamble leads up to my judgment that the financing of hospital and medical care should be universal, comprehensive, and tax-based. People do not choose to be ill and do not want to use health care. The fact of needing health care services marks off individuals as less—not more—fortunate than the rest of the community and, therefore, provides no grounds for exposing them to additional economic burdens as well.

The undesirability of illness and associated health care use holds at any income level; it is not a special situation for "the poor." The wealthy or middle-income individual or family, struck by illness, is thereby made worse off than others at the same income level. This in turn means that the financing system should *not* subsidize only those below a certain income level or in particular categories unless one has specific grounds for regarding some people, or their illnesses or well-being, as simply less important than others. A case for selectivity in principle requires some argument of greater or lesser eligibility for different groups.

In fact, the whole argument is miscast in terms of different groups, of "us" and "them." In a universal system, the community collectively provides for its health care as a sort of consumer cooperative, just as it provides for its own security—internal police and external defense. Individual provision of either is simply less effective and inequitable.

Of course very few individuals actually provide for their own health care, any more than they provide for their own security. The real alternative to universal, public insurance is partial, private insurance, by which subgroups of the population provide collectively for their purchase of care. In either case the funding is a collective process, the only question is the number and composition of the collectives. In principle, one could imagine a situation in which universality could be achieved through a multiplicity of private collectives, with a public insurer of last resort for those not part of any private group. In practice, as U.S. experience clearly demonstrates, multiple-group purchase results in a system that is very far from universal, that is high inequitable, and that is extraordinarily expensive.

People do not choose to be ill and do not want to use health care. The fact of needing health care services marks off individuals as less—not more—fortunate than the rest of the community and, therefore, provides no grounds for exposing them to additional economic burdens as well.

As for the distribution of economic burden in this cooperative enterprise, there is further misleading rhetoric in favor of users paying—occasionally offered in Canada—to the effect that those who can afford to pay should do so. The usual source of such rhetoric is physicians, trying to raise their prices by billing their patients directly. The quick answer is, indeed, those who can afford to pay should do so, and they do. That is implicit in a proportional or progressive tax-based system, in which people with higher incomes pay a larger share of the costs. What does not follow is that at *any* income level, high or low, those who happen to *become ill* should pay more. That is quite a different, and I believe an indefensible, argument.

Once we adopt the perspective that health care is about health and that its utilization, being associated with illness, identifies the user as one struck by misfortune rather than a recipient of "benefits," it seems to me difficult to make any purely principled argument for user-pay finance, or for selectivity and discrimination. The burden of moral argument shifts from the advocates of universal, comprehensive coverage and public finance to those who should presumably offer some grounds for "taxing the sick," or for treating some people's misfortunes as more deserving of collective support than others. At this point, however, it is common to find a second line of attack against universality and/or public finance—the prudential or practical. This argument comes particularly from economists, who are habituated to thinking in terms of trade-offs.

COST CONTROL AS A SUBSTITUTE FOR EFFICIENCY

The argument is that while universal and comprehensive coverage may enhance equity as well as reduce the exposure of individuals to economic risk, such coverage nevertheless induces, in the most extreme form, "moral hazard," "excessive" utilization, and excessive costs. When care is "free," people will use "too much," and costs will be too high. Universality may be equitable, but it is inefficient.

It is therefore necessary, so the argument goes, to balance the desirable features of universal, comprehensive coverage against these undesirable "side effects," in particular through the use of such user-pay features as deductibles and coinsurance. Such features do indeed increase the economic burden on the ill, but without them the utilization and costs of health care would be far too large. Private insurance then finds its justification in offering a range of alternative forms of coverage—again providing scope for consumer sovereignty.

This argument is flawed both logically and empirically. Logically, its proponents define "excessive" use relative to the standard of consumer sovereignty—i.e., what people would choose or be able to use if they were paying full cost—which as noted above is not the standard for appropriate use employed by most of the noneconomist world. Most of us define appropriateness in terms of health outcomes—Is the care likely to contribute to the user's health?—which need not bear any systematic relationship to willingness or ability to pay. So the criterion for excessive use is incorrect in that it rests on a standard of valuation that most of us do not accept.

Secondly, the moral-hazard argument is in application simply a conventional assumption that when a "good" is "free," people will wish to use more of it. Again, the semantic trap of the word "good" has confused the issue. Patient/consumers do *not* want health care for its own sake. It is not a "good." They want it only insofar as they perceive that it will benefit their health. These perceptions, in aggregate, do not necessarily respond to "free" care in the conventionally assumed manner.

The empirical facts do not support the argument either. Intercountry comparisons, particularly between the United States and Canada, but also between the United States and European countries, show that more comprehensive coverage is associated with *better* control of costs—the exact opposite of the "moral hazard" argument. The unfolding of international experience over the last two decades continues to drive home the lesson that cost and utilization expansion is *easier*, not harder, to control in universal and comprehensive systems.

At this point it is important to stress that cost control, *per se*, is an intermediate, not an ultimate, objective. There is much ill-thought-out rhetoric about what countries can and cannot afford, but in fact the real issue is one of priorities. All developed nations could easily spend far more than they now do on health care—*if* they wanted to. Behind efforts to control costs are judgments that the payoffs from increased costs in terms of health improvements are either nonexistent or too small to justify the outlays. Otherwise, cost increases are not a problem at all.

Similarly the very powerful though less publicized efforts to thwart cost control and promote cost expansion, which are mounted by providers in every country, but most successfully in the United States, reflect a strong commitment to the value of increased outlays, either because of their health effects, or, more simply, because all health expenditures translate directly into incomes of providers or other suppliers of goods and services in the health care industry.

Where cost control has been relatively successful, as in Canada, it has operated through two main channels. First, it has controlled the rate of escalation of provider incomes. In Canada this has been achieved by bargaining over uniform fee schedules for physicians and global budgets for hospitals backed up with various forms of industry-specific wage control. The process is contentious and must be continuous, but it does work. Second, capacity constraints are applied—with greater or lesser success—to hospital facilities, beds, and major equipment, and to physician supply. Both the mechanisms and the levels of success vary over regions and time, but the general principle is clear. The escalation of service utilization is controlled through control of the capacity of the system.

In Canada, and in several other countries, there is increasing interest in the possibility that full control may require full global budgeting, for physicians as well as hospitals. This is a logical extension of present policies—using global financial constraints to control costs directly. Such policies share with capacity constraints the underlying assumption about effectiveness—that more utilization, in general, will not yield increased health benefits and that therefore the community will be better off by restraining the flow of resources into this sector.

Indeed, one cannot overemphasize that the adoption of cost control as an objective requires either that one make this assumption or that one assume that providers of health care are overpaid. Conceivably, one could advocate cost control purely on the ground that costs were being driven up by inflated incomes, independently of utilization patterns. While there is clearly some truth in this in particular settings, most observers have focused attention on the effectiveness or ineffectiveness of service patterns.

Control of provider incomes and restraints on physical and workforce capacity have required, where they have been effective, sole-source funding. Universal coverage places the public insurer in the position of being the sole purchaser of care on behalf of the community. Conceivably this single-buyer function could be carried out by a private agency, though this would require very close regulation. But it is hard to see how it is possible to reconcile sole-source control with multiple insurers. The experience of the United States is not encouraging.

One way or another, some single agency has to be able to place a cap on the total number of dollars paid out on behalf of a given population. Perhaps a number of capitated organizations could do this, each controlling outlays for its own population. But Canadian and other experience suggests that such control is extremely difficult, if not impossible, without simultaneous control over the rate of inflow of new capacity into health care. If more and more physicians, and more new and expensive high-tech equipment, keep on coming into the field, global caps on spending will be pushed off. (In principle there is no reason why new technology should not serve to *lower* costs rather than to raise them. In practice, however, even when such savings occur, they are absorbed by an expansion in servicing rates. Otherwise, of course, cost-reducing innovation would threaten the incomes of established providers, and that is rarely permitted to occur!)

In the U.S. context, the implication would appear to be that global budgetary controls must be extended to hospitals, regardless of which insurer is paying the bills, and mandatory and binding fee schedules must be established for physicians. But enforced by whom? Again, both U.S. and international experience confirms what analysis would suggest, that enforcement of financial controls is virtually impossible if one does not control the finances. He who does not pay the piper will have little success in calling the tune. When there are large numbers of small payers, the piper calls the tune.

One approach would be to consolidate and expand Medicare and Medicaid to cover the whole population. Another would be to move state by state. State-based comprehensive coverage would presumably absorb the functions of Medicare and Medicaid, leaving the federal government with the task of regulating, maintaining standards, and supplying funds. Meanwhile, the trend toward self-insurance by private employers should make them more willing to consider state-specific cooperative action, if it could be combined with plausible cost-control features.

What foreign experience does teach, very clearly, is that there is no necessary conflict between cost control and universality. Quite the contrary. Sole-source funding is apparently essential to cost control, even as universality and comprehensiveness are the only approaches ethically consistent with the values held by most citizens of developed nations.

It makes no sense for an external observer to try to tell Americans what is administratively and, perhaps more importantly, politically feasible. The details of new forms of coverage will have to be worked out on the ground, by people familiar with the systems that they will have to modify and extend. But it also makes no sense to continue with multiple and partial public programs, in an environment of even more—and more partial—private programs. In such a situation no one is able to exercise any control over costs and utilization; the only strategy for survival by any one organization is to pass its problems on to someone else, and make them worse in the process.

What foreign experience *does* teach, very clearly, is that there is no necessary conflict between cost control and universality. Quite the contrary. Sole-source funding is apparently essential to cost control, even as universality and comprehensiveness are the only approaches ethically consistent with the values held by most citizens of developed nations. It further follows that most of the current activities of private insurers are in fact very costly make-work—pure wasted effort.

Since this make-work is very well reimbursed, some way presumably will have to be found to buy out these now established stakeholders. Indeed, many of the specious arguments *against* universality come from quarters that lead one to suspect that their authors are quite aware of the potential of universal systems for cost control and improved efficiency— and foresee that they themselves would be the losers!

The problems of organizing gainers from universality and of buying off or outmaneuvring the beneficiaries of the existing system are made more difficult, since by definition, the more expensive a system is, the more people there are who draw incomes from it. The very inefficiency of the U.S. approach creates large and well-established stakeholders in the status quo. But if the difficulty of the task suggests phasing in change, such phase-in must be designed to strengthen, not to weaken, the constituencies for change.

In this regard the traditional U.S. practice of extending coverage to successive groups in turn seems deliberately designed to halt a phase-in process short of completion. Each group that gains coverage loses interest in pushing the process forward for the next group. On the other hand, if one phases in universal coverage for a restrictive class of benefits, as Canada did in providing hospital coverage for the whole population, this raises the obvious logical questions: If hospital coverage, why not medical coverage? Moreover, it shows that universality could work.

One can also phase in by geographic region—province, for example, or state. Again, this approach raises the same questions: If it works there, why not here? The pressures for extension are strengthened. But phase in by population subgroup, like categorical coverage generally, seems to be the equivalent of designed-in failure. When you split your population, you defeat the collective purpose.

THE DELIVERY OF CARE AND THE MAINTENANCE OF QUALITY

"Quality of Care" has been a semantic trap as productive of confusion and deception as the economist's jargon of "goods." Concerns for "quality," real or feigned, are the standard opening riposte to any proposal to limit the escalation of costs or to make any significant changes to the status quo in health care delivery and finance. Yet quality of care, in a fundamental sense, is very far from a trivial or contrived issue; it is at the core of the concept of effective health care. It is important, however, to understand what the issue really is and, equally important, what forms the threats to quality actually take.

First, there is a tendency in some quarters to *define* quality in terms of the total cost of care. On the assumption that "more is better," more and more expensive services and personnel are treated as equivalent to "quality." With this definition, there is of course an inevitable trade-off between cost control and "quality." But the argument is circular; in effect, quality has been defined as cost, so less cost is the same as less quality. This is not very helpful—unless of course one is trying to fight off cost control.

As noted above, cost control for its own sake is a nonsense objective. If that really *were* the objective, the policy would be obvious—shut down the health care system. What is really sought is more effective use of the resources being devoted to health care—more bang for the buck—in terms of health outcomes achieved. The attempts to control escalation are rooted in the assumption, for which I believe there is overwhelming supporting evidence, that in the United States in particular the costs of health can be capped and reduced without any deleterious effects on anyone's health and, indeed, that this would be possible with actual improvements in health.

The arguments for a necessary trade-off between quality and cost control (other than the purely circular ones noted above) tend to slide around this evidence by defining quality, not in terms of health outcomes—which I believe can be the only true test—but in terms of some variant of the consumer-sovereignty principle. Such arguments reduce to the notion that if people are accepting a particular level and pattern of care, whether or not it leads to better health outcomes, that must represent desired care. Utilization becomes its own justification. But very few people voluntarily undergo care that they know to be ineffective. Unnecessary utilization is not a choice but a mistake.

Again, the focus on health outcomes as the objective in health care enables us to cut through such rhetoric and simply pose the question, Could Americans spend less on health care than they do now and still have as good or better health? The answer is, I believe, clearly yes; moreover, if it is not so, then the objective of cost control needs to be rethought.

If there is no necessary threat to quality in a universal, comprehensive, and cost-controlled system, however, it does not follow that the maintenance of quality, in the sense of attainment of good therapeutic outcomes, is automatic. All countries that have moved to a public *payment* system have left in place the basic structure of professional regulation, licensure, training requirements, and professional accreditation and self-regulation, which in one form or another seems universal in the developed world. This structure would, in a system of universal health insurance in the United States, function as well or as badly as it does now.

Universal coverage has no necessary, direct effect on quality of care. It can, however, have several indirect effects. On the positive side, universality ensures access. If no care at all can be considered inferior to some care in most cases, then logically, improving access represents better quality, on average. Too often, the rhetorical issue of quality is posed as if only those who actually receive care should count in the denominator, as if a system that leaves out a large part of the population can still claim to be "high quality" on the basis of the care it provides to those who actually receive it. Once again, defining the objective of the system in terms of its impact on the health of the community clears up this confusion.

Moreover, universality makes possible the creation and use of a comprehensive data base with which to identify and evaluate patterns of care and their outcomes. It has to be confessed that there are few examples of this possibility having been taken up by those countries that have "gone universal," including Canada. An extraordinarily rich resource both for epidemiological and clinical research and for management and control of the health care system has been remarkably little used, partly for political reasons. Nevertheless, the resource is there, and it is slowly coming into greater use.

On the negative side, the control of fees and provider incomes clearly does have an impact on patterns of care and, it is widely alleged, on provider attitudes and satisfaction. In a fixed-fee system, which appears to be the only way to reconcile fee-for-service and cost control, there are strong incentives for short and frequent visits punctuated by procedures, referrals for testing, and prescriptions. Fewer and longer visits, with more time spent by the clinician in simply thinking about the patient's problem and asking questions, might represent a better investment of time. But thinking time is hard to document and reimburse. Providers, in turn, are unhappy with "production-line" medicine, particularly when their incomes rise less fast than they would like even with this style of care.

What is frequently neglected, however, is that these are *not* problems of public, universal systems per se. They will emerge—are emerging—in the fragmented, entrepreneurial United States. One sees increasing complaints in the U.S. medical journals that procedural services are greatly overpaid relative to cerebral services, and the discrepancies seem worse than in Canada. Their causes run deeper than who pays the bill.

Essentially, the problem is that the numbers of providers are rising faster than the population, and the range of technology they wish to deploy is being extended faster than the population wishes to pay for it. If the doctor-to-population ratio keeps rising, then either an ever-larger share of national income must be paid over to doctors (cost escalation), or doctors' incomes, at least in relative terms, must fall. This proposition is not "socialism" but arithmetic. Similarly, if the reach of technology and the professional ambitions of providers are constantly being extended, then again, either costs must escalate or professionals must feel frustrated—again quite independently of the funding system.

Canadian physicians *do* appear to feel unhappy with their financial circumstances and frustrated with what they (although no one else in the country) perceive as an "underfunded" system. But interestingly, their complaint in most cases is not with the universal, comprehensive financing system as such, but simply with what they perceive as not enough money made available for its support. They would be equally unhappy, perhaps even more so, with a system of private coverage that was effective in controlling costs. Insofar as any Canadian physicians find private coverage attractive, it is because they believe, probably rightly, that it is impossible to limit cost escalation in such an environment. If the new competitive medicine in the United States should begin to prove this view wrong, their allegiance will shift rapidly.

The point, then, is that there *are* some real quality issues implicit in a disgruntled medical profession that is unhappy with its income prospects and feeling pressured to practice production-line medicine. But this description could as easily fit U.S. physicians working in a competitive HMO, a for-profit PPO, or any other environment in which an external organization is trying to limit cost escalation. It is in Minnesota, not Canada, that physicians are trying to unionize!

Any effective restriction on cost escalation is going to make physicians unhappy, and such restrictions are, in the long run, inevitable. The objective should be to manage a "soft landing" for the ambitions of the health care sector so as to minimize the negative effects of the adjustment process.

In this regard, it is worth emphasizing that there is no evidence at all that the health of Canadians is suffering in any way from the alleged unhappiness of their physicians. Indeed, there is a good case to be made for the argument that the annual battles over fee schedules that are played out between physician associations and provincial governments provide a symbolic outlet for a good deal of inevitable frustration, in a "safe" and channeled environment with well-known rules. How do American physicians work off *their* fears and frustrations? And what effects does it have on their patients? They have a good deal more to fear than Canadian physicians do. Are there quality effects from this?

The bottom line, I suppose, is that the maintenance of quality is a rather complex process in every health care system, which is far from perfect but on the whole works out a lot better than any obvious alternatives. Universal public coverage does not make the quality-control problem any worse; on the contrary, it generates information and control levers that could in principle improve significantly the degree of quality monitoring by the reimburser. In practice, however, this does not appear to happen—at least not yet.

I have left out of this discussion the whole issue of malpractice and, more generally, the role of the tort system in providing incentives for the maintenance of quality of care, or penalties for its absence. Such an adversarial approach seems, to a non-American, at least wholly inconsistent with the protection of the important therapeutic relationship between provider and patient, as well as being extraordinarily expensive. I suspect its net effects on quality, both by encouraging defensive overservicing and by degrading provider–patient interactions, are negative.

But it is not clear to what extent, if any, litigiousness is affected by the payment system. It may be that removing the financial dimension from the interaction between patient and provider makes the patient less vindictive when something goes wrong—that patients who are not paying their own bills are less inclined to sue. Certainly malpractice is virtually a nonissue in Canada. But there are other differences between the two legal systems, and between Canadians and Americans, which may account for this. It is conceivable, however, that if U.S. legislatures were directly exposed to a larger share of the costs of health care through a more fully tax-financed system, they might be more inclined to explore, and perhaps respond to, the alleged role of litigation in inflating those costs.

THE LOCUS OF SYSTEM CONTROL

The discussion of quality of care has relied on an implicit assumption that providers of care make the critical decisions about how care will be provided, for whom, and under what circumstances. This is, I believe, unavoidable given the nature of health, illness, and medical care, and is not going to change under any conceivable—let alone feasible—funding system. Universal coverage leads to a significant increase in the countervailing power of the funder of care, which in practice seems to have to be one level or other of government.

Some European countries still have an extensive system of nongovernmental, not-for-profit reimbursement agencies; but the pressures of cost escalation are driving them into more and more de facto government control of those agencies. Multiple, closely regulated *Krankenkassen* in Germany, for example, seem to be converging into the equivalent of a public insurance system, but with higher administrative costs.

The consumer has never played a very significant role in controlling the evolution of health care and is unlikely to do so in the future. The strongest advocates of consumer control, apart from economists, have always been those—professionals and others—who were fairly sure that they could control the consumer. Universal coverage with tax-based funding relieves the individual of an unpredictable and capricious economic burden over which she or he never had much, if any, control.

In the "traditional" view of health care, with third-party coverage, if present, largely limited to paying the bills on demand and asking no questions of providers, it was the professional responsibility of providers to represent patient interests as well as their own—and of course they did do so. It was taken for granted, as implied by the very institution of professionalism, that the individual patient was unable to protect his or her own interests and that caveat emptor was a recipe for disaster; this, I believe, was correct and remains so.

But provider representation of patient interests was never perfect; and providers were and are particularly incapable of protecting the *economic* interests of patients, which are in direct conflict with their own. Physicians protect patients, not payers. Nor have traditional private insurers played this role; they served rather to pass through the escalation of costs while taking their percentage in increased premiums on the way by. Public insurance places one or more government agencies in the position of representing the interests of patients—economic as well as, to a much lesser extent, medical. Universal coverage makes that representation effective; fragmentation appears to make it largely impotent.

But the State does not take over the medical system like a sort of medical "Big Brother;" that is merely part of the political rhetoric of medical associations. Instead, there is a continuing conflict of legitimacy between the professional expertise of providers and the political legitimacy of governments representing the community. The tug-of-war is probably permanent, as both sides can legitimately claim to represent some aspect of patient interests. Providers have to share and compete for power and, to some extent, justify its use.

The U.S. situation is most interesting to an outsider because alone among the developed nations it has not moved into this situation of countervailing professional expertise and public authority. Instead, the United States still tries to develop *private* collective organizations capable of countervailing the power of providers and of representing the interests of patients. The work of Alain Enthoven is probably the most thoughtful and completely articulated analysis of how this process might work. In that approach, it is clearly recognized that the *individual* patient cannot and should not be expected to exercise significant direct control over the provision of medical care. But, conceivably, private "sponsors" could serve as consumer representatives, purchasing care from competitive suppliers. Competition among HMOs and PPOs is a less fully worked out version of this same process.

This approach deserves detailed comment, provided elsewhere. Here it suffices to note that it highlights the problems of what group(s) will represent consumer/patients—who cannot effectively represent themselves—and by what mechanisms (professional ethics, political responsibility, market competition) those groups will be held accountable. Second, the market process, while interesting, has not been tried anywhere else, so it has no empirical support. Universal public insurance places principal responsibility on government for competing with professionals to represent patient interests and determine appropriate levels and patterns of expenditure; this has been the approach chosen virtually everywhere else in the developed world.

The sorts of providers who will predominate under public, universal insurance will be those who were in existence when the system was set up. In no country has the shift to public finance been associated with "revolutionary" changes in the delivery system—despite some expressed intentions. Health care delivery has tended to be very conservative, and public insurance has reinforced that conservatism. The great exception, of course, is in the United States, where revolutionary changes in health care delivery *are* alleged to be underway, and the structure of the delivery system is changing rapidly, almost certainly *because* of the absence of universal public coverage.

It appears that it's the inability of the U.S. funding system to limit the growth of overall costs that promotes the rapid and radical changes. If so, change will continue as long as costs continue to escalate, but the result appears to be change without improvement. For our purposes, however, there is no need to spend much time gazing into this crystal ball. Public insurance is consistent with private fee-for-service medical practice, though not with independent fee setting. It is probably not consistent with for-profit hospital operation, unless that can be reconciled with global budget caps.

Contracting for particular services with private, for-profit firms is, however, quite consistent with public insurance. There is no reason why a for-profit laboratory or ambulatory-surgery center should not perform specified services on contract for a hospital or a physician, so long as this is within an overall controlled budget. The combination of for-profit subcontracting with overall full insurance coverage and cost control is an area of active exploration in Canada and the United Kingdom at the moment, and probably elsewhere as well. There seem no logical bars to the combination.

SCOPE OF COVERAGE

"Comprehensive" coverage begs some important questions. Where are the boundaries of hospital and medical care? The Canadian system promises to cover all "medically necessary" care but never defines what that is. Elective cosmetic care seems an obvious exclusion, although even there the boundaries are a bit fuzzy. In practice, the questionable areas have not been quantitatively important enough to cause trouble. Ambulatory psychiatric services reimbursed by fee-for-service, however, have been subject to restrictions, and this is probably necessary in any system. A separate system of community-based clinics with salaried staff backed by a few remaining public mental hospitals exists to serve the chronically mentally ill.

The major problem area is long-term care for the elderly. (For the nonelderly, the long-term care population is both small enough and well enough defined not to pose a large financial problem.) For this group, it is unclear where the boundary is located between health care and functional support. Certainly there seems no excuse for placing upper limits on entitlements for health care coverage in the acute-care system. The whole point of insurance is that it should cover the largest losses, not pass the burden back to the individual when the going gets toughest.

But the dual role of Medicaid, in both reimbursing health care for the ambulatory and episodically ill population and providing long-term institutionalization for the dependent and impoverished elderly, should be split up. The funding of what is clearly health care should be absorbed into a universal system rather than be kept separate and continue to stigmatize the poor with welfare medicine at effectively uncontrollable costs. The funding of long-term care, however, should be organized into a separate system.

This raises an unsolved problem with every funding system. Since long-term care is an extension, in some ways, of the home environment, the user-pay principle is entirely appropriate. Long-term care does not serve primarily to restore health, if it does so at all; rather, it provides an alternative form of food and lodging combined with a greater or lesser degree of health care and/or assistance with activities of daily living. Accordingly, public systems of long-term care charge for this accommodation care. Why, then, should not individuals who can afford it purchase superior accommodations—as obviously they do? And on the other hand, how does one move patients from the "free" public hospital system into long-term care where their accommodation must be paid for?

These problems are not wholly intractable. Like the setting of hospital budgets and the negotiation of fees, they are ongoing difficulties that, by the exercise of effort and intelligence, can be dealt with satisfactorily but will never entirely go away—rather like the problems of everyday life. Since the need for long-term care, however, is inevitably closely associated with limited individual resources, it follows that the provision of such care will always be a significant public charge. This, in turn, will require that access to care be controlled by some sort of formal assessment process as well as appropriate placement. But there is no reason why access to supported care should first require impoverishment, much less spousal impoverishment.

Once again, it is the conceptual framework that is the problem. If public funding is thought of as a residual—as public assistance for the unfortunate, imprudent, or incompetent few who are unable to look after themselves—then "we" who do the right thing and look after ourselves (or die in good time) begrudge the cost and exact harsh conditions on "them." If, instead, we can shift our view of the process to see it as a broader collective enterprise in which "we" are providing for ourselves through the public system and in which public funding is legitimate and normal—not evidence of individual failure—then it becomes possible to do the whole job a lot better. (This shift in perspective will undoubtedly be encouraged if increasing numbers of people, through no fault of their own, find themselves in the "they" category.)

The problems do not become smaller merely by virtue of being shifted to public finance. But it does become possible to organize a better balance of institutional and ambulatory support systems when one agency is paying the bill and when the individual cannot constantly be shifted on to someone else as "not our problem." A public agency may in fact choose to contract out the necessary services to for-profit firms. At the end of the rhetoric, however, evidence is beginning to emerge that, in the case of home care, this is *more* expensive than direct provision, for reasons that seem, in retrospect, plausible. Still, the process of assessment, like the provision of finance, has to remain a public function.

CONCLUSION

It is quite apparent that the foregoing does not constitute a detailed blueprint, even a highly idiosyncratic one, for a U.S. system of health care finance. It is intended, rather, to provide an external perspective on the issue and to highlight certain principles that seem critical to thinking about the problem as well as to comment on a certain amount of international experience in the area.

Most critical, I think, is the perspective. If the health care system is thought of as the set of arrangements whereby a community provides for its health care needs, then the financing system falls into place as a device for mobilizing resources for that purpose, for establishing incentives to motivate people and organizations to provide the appropriate goods and services, and for setting (inevitably as a contentious compromise) the levels of reimbursement for those supplying services. It is inherently a collective enterprise in which the laws of the market have never given much guidance, or at least not much that any civilized community was willing to accept. Nor do they now.

In every developed country outside the United States, a public or quasi-public system of finance—universal or almost so—has evolved or been established to take on these tasks. In none is the result perfect, but nowhere is there any public support for turning back the clock. It seems hard to believe that the United States is uniquely incapable of making a public health care financing system work. After all, the standard represented by the present U.S. system should not be difficult to beat.

REFERENCES

Evans, Robert G. "Health Care in Canada: Patterns of Funding and Regulation." *Journal of Health Politics, Policy and Law* 8 (1): 1–43 (Spring 1983).

_____. *Strained Mercy: The Economics of Canadian Health Care*. Canada: Butterworth, 1984.

_____. "Illusions of Necessity: Evading Responsibility for Choice in Health Care." *Journal of Health Politics, Policy and Law* 10 (3): 439–67 (Fall 1985).

7

ON ROBERT EVANS AND THE CANADIAN MODEL OF UNIVERSAL HEALTH INSURANCE

Alain C. Enthoven

OVERVIEW

Despite superficial appearances to the contrary, the points on which Professor Evans and I agree are far more numerous and important than the points on which we disagree. In particular, I share his criticisms of the conventional thinking of many American health care economists.

We agree that there ought to be a public policy of universal health insurance. While his paper does not focus on the positive reasons, I am sure we agree that medical care responds to a basic human need. Health and health care for the sick are prerequisites to "life, liberty and the pursuit of happiness." Nobody should be denied care that could cure illness, restore function, or relieve suffering because of an inability to pay. Nobody should be subjected to financial hardship because of the cost of care.

We agree that many of the main arguments advanced against universal health care coverage are false. It is not true that such coverage must be inflationary. Health care inflation in the United States is much more the result of the "guild free choice" model of health care finance and of public policies that reinforce the cost-increasing incentives in the system. We could have noninflationary universal coverage. It is not true that out society cannot afford universal coverage. Indeed, a rational system of universal coverage with built-in incentives for economy could reduce costs. Two countries that have universal coverage, Great Britain and Canada, spend substantially lower shares of GNP on health care than we do.

Like Evans, I believe that health care costs are driven by provider behavior and the overall financial incentives and limits in the system. The argument that costs are driven by excess consumer demand caused by free care is false. Most of the cost is spent on the few who are very sick. And doctors make the decisions on resource use for such patients. I don't believe that patients with single vessel disease demand coronary artery bypass grafts from reluctant heart surgeons.

Many of the main arguments advanced against universal health coverage are false. . . . We could have noninflationary universal coverage. It is not true that our society cannot afford universal coverage. Indeed, a rational system of universal coverage with built-in incentives for economy could reduce costs.

Evans and I agree that health care costs ought to be contained because society has other needs that also demand resources. For example, I believe that in our country elementary and secondary education is badly underfunded, and this will be detrimental to the future of our democracy and our economy. Classes are too large, and teachers are underpaid. Although I disagree with some of the wasteful programs and strategies of the Reagan administration, I believe that roughly the present share of GNP is needed for national defense. And we have a huge federal deficit. So something serious must be done to contain the growth in health care spending.

Evans and I agree that a "free market" in health care and health insurance cannot achieve efficiency and equity. Markets for health insurance and health care have too many features that make market failure endemic.

We agree that the only way to achieve equity and cost containment is a rational comprehensive public policy that addresses the whole system. And we agree that, to date, the United States has not adopted such a policy.

THE CANADIAN MODEL FOR THE UNITED STATES?

It is implicit in Professor Evans's paper that the United States ought to adopt the Canadian model of universal health insurance. And in any case, it is a leading candidate, a prominent competitor to my Consumer Choice Health Plan proposal. I think the Canadian model deserves serious discussion. I am not now prepared to write a thorough and detailed essay on this topic. But I will offer my thoughts in outline.

First, Canada has achieved universal coverage. Canada has a federal-provincial system, somewhat analagous to Medicaid in the United States. That is, the federal government offered powerful financial incentives to the provinces to adopt provincial systems of universal coverage meeting federal standards, and the provinces responded. At first, the federal government shared the costs fifty-fifty. Then Canadians came to realize that fifty cents on the dollar left the provinces with too weak an incentive to control costs, so the federal government switched, in effect, to a per capita fixed-dollar contribution (depending on income levels, etc.), leaving the provinces wholly at risk for the marginal costs of their systems. From that time onward, the provinces brought expenditure growth under control.

In great majority, Canadian doctors are in fee-for-service solo practice. Hospitals are paid by provinces on the basis of global budgets prospectively determined. Overall costs are contained by the global budgets in the case of hospitals and by the ability of the provinces to limit the growth in fees paid to physicians.

Thus, the Canadian system is universal and cost contained. From 1971 to 1981, health care expenditures were a constant 7.4 to 7.6 percent share of GNP. The jump to 8.4 percent in 1982, as Evans notes, had more to do with the denominator than the numerator. By contrast, in the United States, health care expenditures rose from 7.6 percent of GNP in 1970 to 9.4 percent in 1980 and 10.5 percent in 1982. Apparently its share is still rising.

I believe that from the point of view of the consumers and taxpayers, a fair appraisal would have to conclude that the Canadian model *is decisively superior to what we have in the United States today.* I do not want to debate Professor Evans on the proposition that the U.S. nonsystem is superior to the Canadian system.

As well as universality and cost-containment, the Canadian system has other features that contribute to the widespread popular approval it commands. For one, in that context, the fee-for-service system gives doctors powerful incentives to be accessible to patients. So, I suppose, access is good, at least in the metropolitan areas. And the simplicity of one payor and one fee schedule per province must create vast savings in paperwork compared with the U.S. system. Just think, the doctor fills out one claim form and sends it to the province! The patient isn't involved in billing and paying. Our comparative shares of GNP do not count the many hours Americans have to spend struggling to figure out their medical bills and filing claims.

In fact, I would conclude that if one considers universality and simplicity to be important, and if one does not believe that the structure and evolution of the delivery system is important, then the Canadian model would be hard to resist.

Still, I am sure Professor Evans would be the first to admit that all is not perfect north of the border. For one thing, the Canadian health care system seems to be even more politicized than ours, if that is possible. And some of the provinces have been experiencing strikes and "job actions" by doctors. I am not worried about the financial condition of Canadian doctors. Canadians are probably still paying substantially more than what would be required to induce a supply of well-qualified persons into medicine (i.e., above-market incomes). But I would be concerned about the quality of care and interpersonal relations if the medical profession is chronically involved in such concerted industrial action.

But more important and fundamental, I see no long-term incentives for improvement in the organization and efficiency of the delivery system in the Canadian model. The enactment of universal health insurance froze the delivery system. It killed the one prepaid group practice that existed in Canada. In the United States we have about twice the acute hospital beds we would need if everyone were cared for by an efficient delivery system. We need to shut down about 40 percent of them. But that just wouldn't happen in a Canadian model. It doesn't happen in Britain, and I doubt it happens in Canada. What Charles Schultze called "the do no direct harm rule" would operate. Government cannot be seen as directly harming individuals. That is why it is next to impossible to shut down an unneeded defense installation or post office. Only the impersonal forces of the market can shut down unneeded facilities. Similarly, we have too many too highly paid specialists in many specialties. We probably have three to five times the number of neurosurgeons we would need in an efficient system. Yet, neurosurgeons are among the highest paid doctors. A Canadian-style model would freeze this in place forever. Only an appropriately structured market in which cost-conscious delivery systems compete to serve cost-conscious consumers has a chance of correcting such imbalances. But if they are not corrected, "cost-containment" won't be the same as efficient delivery of care.

I believe that compared with the fee-for-service solo-practice model, the competing HMO model offers many incentives to improve quality and economy over the long run. Already we see that HMOs use resources differently and, I believe, more efficiently. Compared with uncontrolled fee-for-service plans, they reduce inpatient use considerably and substitute less costly ambulatory care. Comparisons are difficult to make because definitions and customs are not entirely the same. But it appears the Canadians have hospital utilization rates that are much too high. Evans reports Canadians had 1,958 hospital days per 1,000 per year in 1982. The 1983 U.S. figure was about 1,070. (I am sure these data are not strictly comparable. Perhaps Professor Evans can give us a correct comparison.) Quality and economy usually go hand in hand. If a patient is seriously ill, the best and most economical result is achieved if the right diagnosis is made promptly and if the appropriate procedures are done by proficient providers. Capitation financing characteristic of HMOs rewards such quality and economy, and it gives physicians incentives to form cohesive associations that perform peer review. Fee-for-service can reward poor-quality care. I don't see any development in the Canadian system that encourages physicians to work together to improve quality and economy.

I see no long-term incentives for improvement in the organization and efficiency of the delivery system in the Canadian model. The enactment of universal health insurance froze the delivery system.

Quebec officials speak of "*la practique légère*," in which physicians make good incomes by churning easy patients on which the fees per unit of time are good. What incentive is there to solve the patients' medical problems if you can keep seeing them in brief visits?

I don't see what serious incentive Canadian hospitals have to improve quality of care and service, or to introduce cost-reducing innovations such as outpatient surgery centers or home nursing care. They get their money in the form of global budgets from provincial governments, not payments on behalf of satisfied patients. This is bound to take a toll in the long run. What is there to restrain the growth in the length of coffee breaks and other provider perquisites?

An unfortunate but inevitable consequence of a government takeover of any industry is rigidity and provider domination. Canadian officials are concerned about these problems. In Ontario, there appears to be a good deal of interest in Health Service Organizations (HSOs) in which physicians receive incentive payments for reducing the inpatient use of their enrolled populations. But those are far from HMOs. There is no "lock in" and no real incentive for patients to join and stay with their HSO. I have characterized HSOs as "baby second cousins of HMOs."

I think the question of the importance of the evolution of the delivery system accounts for much of the difference in point of view between Evans—and others who support the Canadian model for the United States—and myself. I think incentives and delivery system organization are very important over the long term. But I'll admit nobody is yet able to prove that one or another approach makes any difference for health. I believe that over the long run, we could obtain a much more efficient, flexible, adaptive model in the United States through consumer choice than through a Canadian model.

Would the Canadian model be acceptable in the United States? Political realism and feasibility are very hard to judge. I have seen very experienced senior politicians make judgment calls that proved to be wildly unrealistic. And though I have long experience in government, I cannot claim any special wisdom here. Yet these questions are of fundamental importance, and a serious observer must form opinions about them.

As a universal model for the United States, I believe there is no way the Canadian model would be acceptable. In judging this, I think it is important for citizens of such regulatory-minded states as New York, Massachusetts, New Jersey, and Maryland, as well as people who live and work inside the Beltway, to realize that there are large cultural differences among regions in this country that bear on health care and health care finance. What is and ought to be for New Yorkers really is very different from what is and ought to be as seen by, say, Texans, Californians, or residents of the Rocky Mountain states. A Canadian model might be a reasonable candidate for Massachusetts. Indeed, they are not very far from it. But if Massachussans want it for themselves, they would be wise not to try to force it on Californians and Texans.

American culture generally favors self-reliance, local decisions, private action, pluralism, multiple competing systems, and individual choices. Americans generally prefer these values to centralization and efficiency in public administration. These values are particularly strongly held west of the Mississippi. I think any realistic policy for the United States must take serious account of them and recognize the important fact of cultural diversity. For example, fee-for-service solo practice is the dominant model in New York. Multispecialty group practice is practically unknown. Although more than 1.5 million New Yorkers are in HMOs, the HMO idea seems not to be well-regarded by the intelligentsia and the well-to-do. In

California, over 6 million people are in HMOs and Preferred Provider Insurance is expanding like wildfire. HMOs list among their members many university faculty, scientists, and engineers in high-tech firms. Multispecialty group practice is widespread and widely considered to be a high-quality form of care.

The imposition of the Canadian model on the United States would upset many powerful private interests that would be sure to coalesce to oppose it. Physicians would see it as making the state their paymaster. They could be counted upon to oppose it vehemently, even if society followed the Canadian and British examples and tried to buy them off with high fees initially. Hospitals would divide. The financially weak ones would see salvation in such a scheme. But the strong hospitals who see themselves as winners in the competitive model would oppose it. And they are well represented in the political process. Private insurance companies would see their businesses wiped out, and they are politically powerful. HMOs know what Medicare did to prepaid group practice in Canada. Their arguments would be pretty persuasive. Employers would divide on the issue, but many large ones would likely oppose it in the expectation that taxes on them would pay for other people's employees.

It is interesting to speculate on how organized labor would respond. For the large, powerful, well-paid unions—the UAW, USW, Teamsters, etc.—the Canadian model would have to mean a leveling down in benefits. This country cannot afford universal coverage at the UAW standard and cost. The leaders of these unions would see the end of a valuable bargaining prize; there would be less of an advantage to being in a union. I doubt they would really support the idea. Many articulate people and groups would join with these interest groups in a powerful chorus against "socialized medicine." I do not doubt that some of the more determined leftists in our society would be undaunted by the challenge of ramming it down the throats of the opposition, but that is not the way we do things in our democracy.

I would read the lesson of the Canadian experience in a way other than to conclude we should adopt their model. I believe we cannot achieve universal health care coverage without substantial financial support from the federal government. The states on their own do not have the fiscal resources. We ought to follow the Canadian example in enacting a federal program of substantial subsidies for the purchase of qualified health care coverage by all Americans. In addition, we ought to consider providing federal subsidies to states to encourage them to enact programs of universal health insurance meeting federal standards. But the standards ought to be broad enough to permit wide diversity in concept and organizations. For example, such standards ought to permit substantial premium contributions by the economically self-sufficient so that there will be the opportunity to reward them with the savings from joining an efficient health care plan.

If in that context, New Yorkers want to adopt a Canadian-style model, we in California could have no objection. But we would object strongly to any suggestion that they impose their concepts on California. (Frankly, I doubt the idea would sell in New York.)

My guess is that in such a context, the number of states preferring the Canadian model to the competitive model would be small. And as HMO and other Competitive Medical Plan membership grows in such states as Massachusetts and Michigan, the likelihood of their preferring the competitive model grows.

My critics are entitled to ask "what makes you think a Consumer Choice model is any more feasible politically? We haven't seen a rush of interest groups to support it." Indeed, powerful interest groups oppose some of its key features. But the establishment of a Consumer Choice model would be a much smaller step, much closer to the incrementalism that generally characterizes legislation by the Congress. The key move would be to reform the tax treatment of employer-paid health insurance— to convert today's open-ended subsidies into universal entitlement to fixed-dollar subsidies. While labor and the insurance industry oppose it, it doesn't directly attack their interests. It does so indirectly through incentives and market forces. The reform is rational and fair. Versions of it have been supported in bills introduced by Senators Dole and Durenberger and Congressmen Gephardt, Jones, and Ullman (all of Finance and Ways and Means). Such a move would be far easier for our society to swallow than a Canadian-style model. An equal or actuarially equivalent subsidy to everyone, as an alternative to the present system, could have a powerful appeal as the case for it becomes better understood. And the Consumer Choice model is far more compatible with the American values to which I referred.

COMMENTS ON SOME OF EVANS'S ASSUMPTIONS AND VIEWS

Evans writes, "Finally the U.S. in the 1980s, having adopted a new, competitive strategy of health funding and delivery, has so far shown *more* rapid cost escalation than in the 1970s."

In the early 1980s, important changes occurred that will eventually lead to the destruction of the "guild free choice" model. I am referring particularly to the 1982 enactments of the revised Section 1876 (HMO/ CMP option) in Medicare and AB3480 (enabling Preferred Provider Insurance) in California. But I emphatically deny the suggestion that the United States has tried the competitive model and found it wanting in ability to control costs. For one thing, as of late 1986, only about 30 million of 235 million Americans were in competitive medical plans. For another, the health care economy is still badly polluted by the incentive effects of the open-ended exclusion of employer contributions to health benefits from the taxable incomes of employees. Government pays 40 to 50 percent of the extra cost when upper-income groups choose more costly health plans. Many employers remain on the open-ended system. We cannot say we have tried competition until the great majority of the economically self-sufficient are required to make a fully cost-conscious choice of health plan.

Incidentally, Evans's ascribing the post-1983 drop in hospital utilization entirely to the Medicare prospective payment system (PPS) ignores the fact that hospital admissions and lengths of stay for those under 65-years-old declined steadily from 1981 to 1985. There is a lot more than PPS at work here.

I do agree in general with Evans's view of "the painful prescription" (Aaron and Schwartz 1984).

"Demographic pressure" on health care spending resulting from aging may not be large in relation to economic growth. Moreover, a substantial part of the increased cost with age, as Evans notes, is the cost of dying. As people live longer, age-specific costs may be reduced by that factor.

Still, I think the increasing ratio of retired to working-age population will be an important factor. The trustees of the OAS and DI trust funds note that the ratio of covered workers to beneficiaries fell from 5.1 in 1960 to 3.3 in 1985 and is projected to fall to 2 by the middle of the next century. That means there will be fewer workers to support each retiree.

As Evans notes, a universal publicly financed system need not be more expensive. And future technological developments may be expenditure-reducing as well as cost-reducing, especially if guided by incentives that reward adoption of cost-reducing technologies. As Evans says, "one cannot assert a priori that the effect on costs must be upwards."

I agree with Evans's views regarding the efficacy of coinsurance at the point of service as long-term strategy for cost control. But I think cost consciousness at the time of annual choice of comprehensive health care financing and delivery plans is a very different proposition.

CONCLUDING COMMENT

If I had to boil it down to one point, I would rest my case for the competitive model, in preference to the Canadian model, on the long-term prospects for efficiency-enhancing innovation.

I see great opportunities for innovation in a market-driven system for the following reasons.

1. We need to sort out which are the most efficient and acceptable models mixing multispecialty group practice, for quality and economy, with dispersed primary-care sites for ease of access.
2. We need a great deal of experimentation and empirical tuning of methods of physician payment to find ways of encouraging productivity and quality of service as well as effectiveness and economy in use of resources. While I frequently criticize uncontrolled, unattenuated fee-for-service systems, I do recognize a fee-for-service component may be very important in rewarding doctors for working hard and being attractive to patients.
3. As mentioned earlier, we need large adjustments in facilities and personnel to bring resources used into balance with the needs of the population.
4. We need evolution and development of private-sector methods of quality control.
5. We need innovations in design of coverages to blend the strengths of the HMO model with the advantages of Preferred Provider Insurance to adapt to special needs, such as those of retirees who spend different seasons in different geographic areas and families with children away at school.
6. We need a long-term process of cost-reduction through adoption of more cost-effective technologies and management methods.
7. We need to use market forces to bring provider incomes down to the levels no higher than those needed to elicit an adequate supply of well-qualified persons.
8. We need competition to motivate high quality combined with willing provision of service and ease of access.
9. We especially need innovation and development of concepts of comprehensive care for the frail elderly that enhance their ability to live independently and maximize their ability to care for themselves as an alternative to institutionalization. We are exploring this in the "Social HMO" experiments.

The Canadian and British models, for all their strengths, are frozen. They lack the incentive and ability to evolve to better meet society's needs.

The British find it extremely difficult even to close inefficient hospitals when a consolidated regional replacement hospital is in place. I wonder how the Canadians are doing in relocating hospital capacity with changing needs.

Expenditure containment should not be confused with cost reduction. The health care financing and delivery system should be designed so that its providers and managers have powerful incentives to minimize the total social cost of illness and its treatment. Cost containment that simply shifts costs to untreated patients is not real cost control. I am sure the British system achieves a part of its low percent of GNP by such cost shifting. There is a very real cost when a patient with a painful arthritic hip is kept waiting two years or more for a hip replacement. It does not show up on the GNP accounts, but it is not zero. (The waiting lists in the English National Health Service are not an American rhetorical fantasy. The College of Health in London publishes a guide to waiting lists.) Over the years, I think we should watch this aspect of the Canadian system.

REFERENCE

Aaron, H., and W. Schwartz. *The Painful Prescription*. Washington, D.C.: Brookings Institution, 1984.

8

FORGING THE AGENDA

Shelah Leader
Marilyn Moon

Debate about the future of health care in the United States often focuses on marginal tinkering with the payment for and delivery of care. Major changes often result only in responses to unplanned or unanticipated forces such as inflation or technological change. Mindful of this criticism of the formulation of health policy, we sought to examine the health care system as a whole and then strategically consider what, as an association, we thought the overall goals should be. Such discussion could then help shape our incremental policy proposals as well.

Since our experts and AARP leaders and staff deal with the everyday policy debates, remaining focused on the big picture was not always an easy task. Practicality and political realities were often raised as sobering influences during our exchanges. Indeed, implementation rather than goals generated most controversy. This brief essay attempts to convey a flavor of the two-day meeting attended by the experts and AARP volunteers and staff as well as to suggest our reactions and conclusions as participants. Rather than provide a strict chronological account of the discussion, we have imposed a structure post hoc. A transcript of the proceedings supplied the exact quotations and helped us reevaluate our own notes and impressions. Participants in this discussion are identified in the introduction and list of contributors to this book.

Although we sought to bring together individuals with differing perspectives, there was considerable agreement on the major goals for reforming our health care system. Broadly speaking, the goals for a new health care system can be divided into these three categories:

1. Universal coverage of a uniform package of benefits
2. Improvements in how care is delivered
3. Increased attention to the quality of care

More lively debates ensued over how best to achieve these goals. Again the discussion can be thought of in these three parts:

1. Who should be in control?
2. Should change be incremental or immediate?
3. What role could an organization like AARP play?

THE GOALS

Perhaps the least controversial discussions surrounded the goal of including everyone in some form of insurance coverage. Regardless of the differences in other areas, the experts all advocated, in brief opening statements, as Enthoven put it, "wall-to-wall universality."

Universality and Uniformity

Early discussion focused on the unacceptability of the gaps in our current health care system. Several of the AARP members put themselves firmly on the conference record in support of addressing the needs of Americans of all ages, not just our oldest ones.

Clarice Jones: I think it is AARP's business to make others aware of our concern for generations coming after us, not just for ourselves.

Also linked to the universal-coverage question was whether this could be accomplished by a patchwork system—a theme that also became part of the implementation of the goals. Nonetheless, the structure of the health system was viewed as such a basic issue that it could not be theoretically separated from the question of universality.

Barbara Herzog: Alain Enthoven's system does not contemplate immediate universality of insurance coverage. If you pay a 40 percent subsidy, what happens to people who decide they can't afford coverage even with that subsidy or who don't want to pay for it?

Alain Enthoven: I will grant you that if you have a system that involves individual choice and people have to sign up, then some people—undocumented aliens or those with different lifestyles—will choose not to sign up. We'll always have providers of last resort such as county hospitals. We'll have to automatically enroll people who don't sign up.

Although the question of who will be covered was rather quickly answered, the discussion of whether there is a minimum set of services or insurance benefits to which all Americans should be assured access generated more controversy.

Shelah Leader: Do I understand that the Canadian system does not ration very expensive procedures, but basically whatever can be done will be paid for by the Canadian system?

Robert Evans: The rationing takes place through the decision on where to site particular facilities and how many to put in place. You do the control through the capital-budgeting side—how many pieces of equipment you will pay for. If they want to buy new equipment, they have to go and get separate approval for that.

Shelah Leader: Very often universality in the U.S. means everybody being guaranteed minimum benefits while cosmetic or expensive procedures would then be rationed or made available through the private sector.

Robert Evans: Cosmetic surgery is not covered in Canada. Where is the borderline where you are repairing a person in a car accident or pinning the ears back on a kid? In the car accident case it is covered, and in the ears it is not. As far as the very expensive procedures are concerned, the principle there is subject to the constraint of how much capacity you are providing. Yes, we will provide the expensive services providing we think they are effective.

The question of first- and second-class care was also discussed.

Robert Evans: We don't seem to mind if the rich go first class, as long as they don't get on a different aircraft. I don't know how to separate amenities from outcomes. If you allow the provider to get different amounts looking after different kinds of folks, you'll get a division of ultimate outcomes.

John Rother: Obviously everyone has to be on the same plane; but where is the plane going? We have to define the basic benefit package. Should it be a minimum that is supplemented by the rich, or should everyone be entitled to everything like Canada?

Robert Kane: Politically and administratively we are locked into a system of financing and delivery. The challenge is to get as much universality and control out of a mixed system as possible. What I would do is build in uniform benefits, uniform choices with a mixed system of care. I believe in universality and in giving everyone a ticket to ride the same plane. I really worry about consigning whole groups of people to public hospitals or cut-rate HMOs. The nice thing about everybody flying on the same plane is that you have the same probability of going down, no matter what section you're in. The differences are in amenities, not fundamental issues.

Alain Enthoven: I agree with about 99 percent of what Bob Kane said. I've been talking about business-class care. I'd like the government to pay for the poor to get into the same delivery system so that from a financial point of view we appear the same to the doctor.

Tom Nelson: I don't think we should talk just about an airplane. We should talk about the bus as well. By that I mean we should talk about access to low technology, like care for Alzheimer's patients.

Karen Davis: I think there is a fair agreement that benefits ought to cover hospitalization and all medically necessary physician services, and there should be no arbitrary limits on quantity. The disagreement centers on how to pay for it.

An Improved Delivery System

Although at several points in the discussion individuals spoke about ideal delivery systems, much of the debate centered on the practical problems facing the existing health care system. The fee-for-service model and a more managed care system such as health maintenance organizations (HMOs) were contrasted. In many cases the focus was on the financial aspects of these two systems rather than on the actual care delivered. These systems were advocated more for their abilities to control costs or simplify beneficiary billing. For example, one exchange among AARP members and staff began with the following observation:

Clarice Jones: I want to share what I've observed in Michigan. My own unhappiness is with the carrier's poor performance. The explanation of medical benefits is indecipherable and is delayed so long you forget what it was all about.

Frank Forbes: We surveyed our members, and 90 percent of them are Medicare recipients. They complain about claims processing, delays, and the paperwork.

Eugene Lehrman: I agree that the carrier is the brunt of our concern. On the other hand, the complaints about coverage and bills disappeared in Madison, Wisconsin, when people enrolled in HMOs.

Anne Harvey: While we do hear that people are unhappy about Medicare's coverage, claims denials, and the confusing paperwork, we're not getting thousands of letters and phone calls from our members demanding that we change the system. The majority of AARP's members are Medicare beneficiaries, and they aren't out to abolish the system.

Bette Mullen: I think whatever model we come up with could generate a lot of flak because it's better to have the devil you know than the devil you don't know. I suspect a lot of our members would be very unhappy with throwing out the system.

Discussion of improvements in the type of services offered centered on the long-term care arena. Participants recognized that this area is much less well developed than the acute-care side. And, in particular, the lack of home- and community-based care was considered at some length. Again, there was a great deal of agreement that such services were needed.

John Rother: We do ask a sample of our members each year what they would change if they could change Medicare, and for the past few years, the leading response has been the desire for benefits to cover home health care and nursing home care. But the answers to those questions are very strongly correlated with education and income. Higher-income folks are much more likely to want to see specific benefits to cover out-of-pocket expenses like drugs, hearing aids, and things they could pay for out of their monthly income.

AARP volunteers were asked what they would do first as part of a long-range reform plan, and they agreed that their first priority would be long-term care for all age groups.

Clarice Jones: We are concerned about generational problems, and this option would make others aware of our concern for generations coming after us, not just for ourselves.

There was general agreement that home care should be included in the long-term care benefit. More controversial was the extent to which long-term care could be tackled at the same time and in the same system as acute care. Here the crux of the issue became the problem of integrating social concerns into a medical model. Participants were generally skeptical of turning this area over to the medical establishment.

Quality

The third goal for improving our health care system centered on quality. Again, this was a relatively noncontroversial goal, but it was not easy to reach consensus on how to achieve that end. While there was no disagreement over the proposition that there must be a quality-control mechanism that aggregates and examines epidemeological data—provider batting averages—there was no clear consensus on how to actually implement an effective quality-control program. Leaving quality judgments up to individual consumers was rejected out of hand. And there was broad support for Robert Kane's assertion that quality should be measured in terms of outcomes.

Robert Evans: I want effective care, but as an ordinary guy, I don't read the *New England Journal of Medicine*, and my idea of effective care is what my doctor says. The answer isn't to educate consumers to second guess their doctors.

Alain Enthoven: There is a lot of truth in that. Information works on providers rather than on consumers. But ever since Florence Nightingale proposed that we keep a public track record on providers, the medical profession has blocked information on who is doing a good or bad job. The medical profession is not interested in the quality of care. Quality for most doctors is how much you pay them.

IMPLEMENTATION OF REFORM

One of the challenges to the four experts invited to the meeting was to offer a viable health care plan for the United States. Rather than just talking principles, we asked Davis, Enthoven, Evans, and Kane to propose a system in as much detail as possible. About two-thirds of the two-day session focused on the steps necessary to achieve some of the goals described above.

The Structure of a Reformed System

With the exception of Robert Evans, who remained enthusiastic about the advantages of his comprehensive public Canadian system, the experts reiterated the need for a mixed system. Nonetheless, the option of a fully public system was raised at an early point in our discussion.

Shelah Leader: If health care is something everyone should have, why don't we think of health care as a public utility—like education, garbage collection, and sewers—and provide and pay for it in the same way?

Alain Enthoven: You can't compel the willing provision of high-quality services, so some cities competitively bid garbage-collection contracts. Maybe we could contract for health services and switch if we're not satisfied after two or three years. We have got this employment-based system, and it is going to be very hard to change it. It has many defects, but it is there and dug in, and it is more realistic to try to work with that and remedy its defects and make sure the people left out of that get taken care of as well than it is to campaign to abolish it.

While there seemed to be some consensus that a mixed approach relying upon the government and employers was necessary, dissatisfaction was expressed about the strength of the providers in controlling the current health care system. Some general comments were also directed at reimbursement reform for the purpose of controlling costs. But Robert Evans challenged the notion of achieving true cost control under a mixed system without strong central control.

Robert Evans: The problem is you can't trade off physicians and hospitals the way you can with garbage collection. The capital and manpower are too highly specialized. In the end, everyone will get a contract. So how do you motivate providers to do a good job? The Canadian experience shows that the public utility does not have to be provider dominated. The government of Ontario responded to the needs of consumers and defeated a doctors' strike over mandatory assignment.

John Rother: We have relevant public opinion data on this subject. The public feels very strongly that employers should be responsible for providing health coverage for employees. The public responsibility is limited to those who are unemployed, retired, and poor.

This led to a debate about whether a mixed private/public system can achieve uniformly high-quality care with effective cost control. Evans insisted that only a universal system with global budgeting can control costs, while Enthoven pointed out that the public-utility approach in England has resulted in an inefficient system characterized by delays and poor care for lower-class people.

Finally, a great deal of the discussion surrounding control of the system and the practical problems to be encountered centered on long-term care rather than on acute care.

Robert Kane: My proposal is essentially the great reformation. We have paid too much attention to orthodoxy in long-term care when there is little evidence to support it. I want to change the payment system and base it on measurable outcomes. Some sort of public-utility model is the best way to provide services that produce benefits, including satisfaction. And we provide a gatekeeper.

Alain Enthoven: I'm not proposing anything for long-term care. I do agree with Karen [Davis] that Medicaid is a very inadequate substitute for a social insurance program. I really don't believe the private sector can come up with a satisfactory financing system, and we do need to have some broad-based mandatory social insurance to pay for it. Bob's [Robert Kane's] idea makes a lot of sense to me. I think these social services should have some kind of a territorially based social model.

Karen Davis: I recommend setting up a new part of Medicare to cover long-term care service including nursing home care, home-help and day-hospital care, and personal and chore services based on the Norwegian model. I'd finance it with a mandatory income-related premium paid by beneficiaries, and there'd be some cost sharing up to a ceiling.

John Rother: Steve Brody has proposed linking reimbursement with limits on activities of daily living. Alternatively, people in the disability community want vouchers so they can hire and fire their own help. That's an interesting thought.

Robert Kane: The California experience with a voucher program showed that there are enormous quality problems. And if you tie long-term care to functional ability, half of those who need care would be ineligible. In general, I agree with Karen [Davis], but I get nervous about linking long-term care with Medicare because it is a medically dominated model.

Incrementalism Versus Rapid Change

While the group accepted the need for major changes in our health care system, debate was lively over the speed of such changes. In large measure, the specter of costs and the current budgetary problems of the federal government cast a note of pessimism over the discussion. Again, the group moved quickly from discussing the ideal into grappling with the political realities. Karen Davis was the most outspoken advocate of incrementalism and had built such a system into her blueprint for change that participants had read.

Jack Christy: I like Karen's incremental approach. If we pile responsibilities onto employers, maybe they'll say, "Who needs all this trouble?" and maybe they'll support a universal program.

Participants were troubled by the reality that, for political reasons, a massive and immediate shift in funding is difficult to sell. But, Davis's incremental approach to change—while politically expedient—may be ineffective in the long run because it will not produce the sizeable payoff in savings and satisfaction needed annually to motivate additional reform over many years. As Evans pointed out, each year that we defer bringing *all* health expenditures into line with the consumer price index, we lose savings at an annual compound rate. If one only factors into the political equation the expected first-year savings, it doesn't seem worthwhile to undertake comprehensive reform. The initial increased outlays from a comprehensive system are more than offset five to ten years later.

Robert Evans: Only if you bite the bullet will you consolidate your political base in support of sweeping changes. You only have a few windows of opportunity to create political changes.

But Karen Davis was skeptical about that approach and persisted in advocating incremental change. She pointed out that if savings are generated quickly, they get built into the Congressional Budget Office's (CBO's) base and are not credited to politicians in future years. She felt that public support would erode over time, as people would ask, "What have you done for me lately?"

In the short term, Enthoven proposed improvements in the HMO rules, such as a coordinated, annual open-enrollment period for all HMOs and intermediate Medicare sanctions for abuse. He also suggested that AARP gather data from its members about good and bad providers in order to create market pressures.

But Evans retorted that so few Americans are enrolled in HMOs that the marginal benefits Enthoven proposed would be insignificant. Instead, Evans thought, mandating physician assignment would yield larger results in savings.

Alain Enthoven: If you try to get mandatory assignment through Congress, you will have a very long twilight battle with the medical profession that probably can't be won. The solution lies in a quote from the president of the California Medical Society, "We were so busy fighting socialized medicine that we got blindsided by capitalism."

That is, Enthoven believes competitive pressures for market shares by HMOs can hold down costs, raise quality, and provide a vehicle for enrolling everyone in the delivery system.

While the attendees saw some merit to Enthoven's approach, they were skeptical that known abuses by HMOs toward poor and elderly enrollees would be effectively curbed by designated sponsors of these groups. Essentially, there was a strong belief that the care offered to Stanford University professors might not be duplicated elsewhere.

All the participants agreed on the importance of providing universal access to a minimum benefit paid for by a progressive tax, but the main stumbling block to achieving this goal was initially raising additional revenues in an era of budget deficit and Gramm-Rudman.

As economists, the experts agreed that net expenditures for universal health care coverage would increase only a relatively small amount, perhaps $10 billion, if universal coverage of a minimum benefit were provided. What would really occur would be a transfer in the amount of roughly $40 billion from the private to the public sector, which would be depicted by the CBO as an expenditure *increase* because CBO ignores private dollars.

That is, Enthoven pointed out, we presently provide tax subsidies for employer-provided health insurance for the wealthy, but the value of that subsidy does not appear in the federal budget as an expenditure. Davis insisted that eliminating the subsidy and providing direct funding for universal benefits would be perceived as a growth in federal spending.

Despite the group's skepticism about coming up with a comprehensive acute-care program that could be implemented rapidly, the discussion on long-term care fared somewhat better. The AARP volunteer leaders, in particular, expressed considerable concern about the need to move as soon as possible in this area. And when the discussion turned explicitly to the question of whether we should tackle the acute-care sector first, the group rejected putting long-term care on the back burner.

Marilyn Moon: Does long-term care have to wait?

Karen Davis: I don't think it can wait.

John Rother: It is hard to sell in the political marketplace something that could be mischaracterized as everybody having a maid. So what are the values we are trying to protect? One is simply the value that people should not have to end their lives without dignity and independence. Another value, which is somewhat separate, is financial protection for families that have a chronically ill member.

While there was broad agreement on the need for long-term care, there was some concern that we presently lack an effective delivery system to prudently manage an expanded benefit. Robert Kane stressed the importance of developing a good case-management system that links chronic and acute care before we inject additional money into nursing homes. This implicitly became another argument for incrementalism, but it represented the only major doubt expressed about the need to rapidly create a public long-term care insurance program.

The Role of AARP

Peppered throughout the two-day meeting was discussion concerning the role of consumer groups such as AARP. How much of the burden for assuring quality and educating consumers should fall on these groups? What other roles might they play? Alain Enthoven, in particular, stressed the role of consumers, especially in a competitive system such as the one he advocates.

Alain Enthoven: Organizations like AARP could get behind the release of more and better quality information. It doesn't take every consumer reading medical journals to create the feeling among providers that somebody is watching them and collecting information on them.

Barbara Quaintance: I wanted to raise the idea of a consumer education program. I think it has its place, although it's not a panacea. It may put pressure on providers for a while, but if consumers don't use the information, that pressure will go away.

But Robert Kane expressed more skepticism in relying on empowering consumers with information.

Robert Kane: We have tremendous variations in practice and in what is accomplished. We would be better off looking at the results of care. We need a different system of accountability. If we move toward a competitive strategy, we don't want providers to compete on the basis of advertising.

The role of consumer organizations in promoting change was also discussed. Are consumers motivated to seek a change in the system? Do they need more information to understand the possible consequences of further change?

John Rother: We should be honest with the American public and tell them you have to spend money to save money.

Robert Evans: The first thing your educational campaign has to do is get away from the notion that somehow the elderly population is a threat to the system. It is not demography; it is the way the health care system is applied. Aging is not antisocial. Individuals aren't dumb, they're caught up in a dumb system.

George Engelter: As a beneficiary I have no quarrel with Medicare. My quarrel is with the forces that are acting on Medicare and causing my Medigap premium to go up a sizeable amount. There is nothing I can do about it. I have to pay.

Gwen Bedford: I don't agree there's no way to get at what the dissatisfaction is. I think there is a great deal of it out there, and I think we should tackle it head on.

Shelah Leader: Sometimes it's misleading to assume that people communicate their discontent. We have to take into account fatalism, like George's reaction to his rising insurance premiums. You can create revolutions by making people aware that their individual problem is indeed a national problem that is remediable. AARP could launch a public education campaign and say there is a better way to run a system.

Barbara Quaintance: People's expectations are so low, they're happy with what they get. We set up a hot line, and our callers don't know what to ask. If people understood what the real problems are, we'd have a different situation to deal with.

Barbara Herzog: How can consumers drive change? In my informal Thanksgiving poll of seven elderly relatives, not one knew what DRGs are. We have to distinguish between unhappiness with Medicare's coverage and dissatisfaction with health care in general. A lot of people confuse the two.

Anne Harvey: Since we've never offered the public a very informed choice, how can we know what they really want? If we're going to mobilize our 25 million members [28 million in 1988], then we have to educate consumers and find out what they really want.

Alain Enthoven: You don't get a revolution without rising expectations. You have to educate people that there is a better system.

Finally, a number of individuals cited the creativity that many have shown in the health care area and the importance of encouraging both formal and informal efforts. Participants felt it was critical to involve states and individuals in an education program.

Gwen Beford: I want to bring out the value of self-help groups, particularly for the care of Alzheimer's and Parkinson's patients. One of the things these groups need is clerical support. No one has bothered about them, but they're an excellent source of respite care and moral mutual support. One self-help group came up with the idea of an apartment building for Parkinson's and Alzheimer's patients so they could support each other.

Eugene Lehrman: Society didn't just stumble upon some of the creative solutions to problems. They were clearly thought out. It's not by chance that in Minnesota they have more nursing home beds than the national average, and the second place goes to Wisconsin. We refer to those two as socially conscious states.

Our state initiated a program called community options. When someone applies for a nursing home, he is assessed, and a plan is drawn up with options for community-based care. It is a system financed by the state. If you are able to, you have to contribute to the cost of home care services. It is targeted on keeping people in their homes.

CONCLUSIONS

What then, if anything, could we conclude from the two days? A lot of questions did remain unanswered, and a lot of problems were put on the table for further discussions at a later date. For example, no strong consensus emerged on the critical issue of whether a basic HMO-type strategy was the appropriate delivery mechanism; no firm answers emerged on how to coordinate acute-care and long-term care goals; and no firm strategies emerged for implementing change.

Nonetheless, we did make considerable progress toward agreement on basic goals, and we did define more clearly the scope of the problems facing us in improving the health care system. Many of the participants felt we had achieved the overall goal of taking a broader look at the system so that our incremental policy decisions in the near future will be better informed. Moreover, an informal poll of the group did result in consensus on the following three concrete priorities:

1. Comprehensive long-term care benefits must be made available to all ages. Expanded benefits should be progressively financed by all taxpayers—not just the elderly. To achieve this goal, we need to launch a public education campaign and mobilize political support for improved long-term care coverage.
2. Everyone must have insurance coverage for all medically necessary hospital and physician services, long-term care—including home care—and limited mental health services.
3. Mandatory assignment of physicians' bills under Medicare to alleviate the major sources of beneficiary discontent with Medicare.

9

NOTES OF A CATSKINNER: ALTERNATIVE FUTURES FOR AMERICAN HEALTH CARE

Robert G. Evans

The principal task of this paper is to provide a commentary and critique of the paper prepared by Karen Davis (hereafter KD) for the AARP seminar on the future of the U.S. health care system. Such a critique, however, would be much less useful and in fact seriously incomplete if it were restricted only to the KD paper. The other two papers by Alain Enthoven (AE) and Robert Kane (RK) are in important respects complementary to KD, such that taken together they provide a more comprehensive survey of issues and policy alternatives.

COMMON VALUES

Furthermore, despite their seemingly radical differences in policy recommendations and in their visions of the appropriate institutional framework for the funding and delivery of health care in the United States, it turns out on closer examination that they all share a common underlying philosophical basis or set of fundamental value judgments about what a community or society should expect its health care system to achieve. (This commonality of view about ultimate objectives or criteria for a "good" system came out even more strongly in the workshop itself.) The marked differences in institutional and policy recommendations represent different choices of means to remarkably similar ends, resulting from different judgments about political and organizational feasibility and different emphases on the significance and severity of various generally recognized problems.

In particular, there was agreement among all presenters that the organization, funding, and delivery of health care was a collective problem for the community as a whole that could not and would not be effectively addressed by isolated individuals acting on their own in some form of market system through unregulated voluntary exchange processes. While the three papers held out very different visions of the appropriate institutional structure, each nevertheless envisioned or recommended a system of *collective* institutions within a tight network of public regulation. The key institutions might be private or semi-private bodies—KD's private employers and insurers under mandate, AE's closely regulated "sponsors," or RK's geographically based public agencies that bear some similarity to the health care systems of the Canadian provinces. The idea that individual "consumer/patients" were or ever could be the principal directors of the behavior of the health care system was dismissed by all concerned.

This is not to say that there is no role for decision making by individual patients, much less that their views and preferences should be ignored. There was general agreement that the present U.S. system should be modified to expand the scope for individual decisions. The papers placed different emphasis on this possibility and suggested different ways of bringing it about. But the chimera of a genuine, unregulated, "free market" in health care, with each consumer/patient making his or her own decisions as to what medical or hospital services to buy, and from whom, at prices determined either by direct negotiation or through open competition among competitive providers was regarded as so totally impractical, on any number of grounds, as to be of interest only to theoretical economists.

Professions and professionals, acting on behalf of patients, not only exist but have a reason for existing. They protect the vulnerable interests of patients who as individuals confronting the health care system frequently have neither the information nor the resources to protect themselves and may be in no physical or emotional state to do so. All the papers, however, reflect the view that providers are not in a position to do an adequate or complete job protecting patient interests in terms of either health or finances and are particularly ill-adapted to protecting collective, as opposed to individual, interests. (Indeed many professionals would reject the idea that they had a duty to do so.) Consequently, the papers propose alternative institutional structures—alternative collective agents acting on the patient/consumer's behalf—to manage the relationship between provider and patient in a more satisfactory manner.

Satisfactory defined how? Again I think that there was a high degree of underlying consensus on ultimate values or principles among the papers, although very different emphasis on what were the most serious questions of the moment. I think that each of the three American authors could comfortably subscribe, in general terms, to the opening declaration of the *Canada Health Act* of 1984, consolidating and making more specific the earlier federal statutes that established the universal public hospital and medical insurance systems in Canada.

> It is hereby declared that the primary objective of Canadian health care policy is to protect, promote, and restore the physical and mental well-being of residents of Canada and to facilitate reasonable access to health services without financial or other barriers.

This leaves plenty of room for debate about definitions and criteria as well as about the major question on which the papers do profoundly disagree—the most appropriate institutional framework for pursuing that very general policy goal. But the underlying consensus on ultimate objectives at least rules out a still more fundamental conflict of values, which is apparent if the present collection of papers is contrasted with the policy proposals of those who apply to health care the unmodified ideology of the "free market."

From that alternative ideological standpoint, the proper objective of health policy is indistinguishable from that of economic policy generally, which is to ensure that, as far as possible, people receive the goods and services that they as individuals—unfettered by public regulation or subsidy—are willing and able to pay for. The variable state of their information, health, and financial resources does not enter as a consideration.

Stated in this bald form, the application of the pure "free market" ideology to health care has relatively few supporters, even in the United States. But the underlying framework—in a fuzzy and only partially understood form—frequently emerges as motivating policy proposals in health care that only make sense in terms of an ideology that holds that the purpose of the health care system is to respond, not to the health needs of patients, but to the dollar-backed market choices of consumers. Private, for-profit firms in competitive markets are extremely good at doing the latter and relatively ill-adapted to the former; not surprisingly, the public rhetoric of their spokesmen often urges the latter—with various forms of enteric coating—as the proper objective of health policy.

In the papers prepared for this workshop, there was little or no overt or disguised conflict over fundamental ideologies; there was, however, a great deal of healthy and constructive disagreement and debate over alternative means for approaching the objectives shared by most members of any humane and civilized society—even including the United States.

COMPLEMENTARITY—DAVIS AND ENTHOVEN

The most apparent complementarity of approach is between the papers by Karen Davis and Alain Enthoven. Superficially, they appear diametrically opposed in approach. KD concentrates on extending insurance in a rather traditional manner to cover the whole population with a more comprehensive and complete range of services while she devotes markedly less attention to how the services will be delivered, by whom, and at what cost. Her principal concern is to promote access for those who now lack it and to spread the associated economic burdens more equitably across the population, from the weaker to the stronger shoulders. In economic jargon, she places a heavy emphasis on the demand side.

AE by contrast devotes most of his attention to the supply side (i.e., the organization and provision of care). He proposes a radical transformation that will improve the efficiency of the delivery system, holding down its costs while improving its effectiveness and controlling the incomes of providers to the benefit of patient/consumers. In this supply-side analysis, relatively little attention is given to how coverage can be extended, either to more people or to more services—though AE recognized the desirability of universal and comprehensive coverage, just as KD recognizes the need for efficiency and cost control.

Davis's Goals, Criteria, and Policy

The KD paper has a particularly logical structure, beginning with a set of goals for health policy, then proposing a set of criteria to evaluate strategies for goal achievement, and finally, proposing a specific policy or set of policies—changes in funding and regulatory structures—most appropriate for the pursuit of the goals.

The specific goals proposed are

1. reduction of preventable morbidity and mortality
2. enhancement of quality of life through maintenance of functional capacity, relief of pain and discomfort, and control over lifestyle

3. assurance that no one is denied access to care because of inability to pay
4. equitable distribution of financing burdens
5. control of health costs by promoting efficient and effective provision of care
6. maintenance and enhancement of quality of care and progress of technology
7. preservation of freedom of choice by patients as individuals or collectively in determining the pattern of their own forms of care

Taken together, this is a formidable set of objectives, though no one could disagree with the desirability of each individually. But as KD recognizes, these goals are to some extent in conflict. The very essence of professional regulation, for example, is radical violation of freedom of choice in alleged protection of quality of care. The claim may be to a considerable extent true, but the conflict is no less real. The problem of quackery suggests that freedom of choice is also in conflict with goals 1 and 2, pertaining to health status. Do we want individuals to be free to choose, and have access to, forms of care generally known to be useless or even harmful?

Indeed, goal 7 is even internally inconsistent. KD makes the very important statement that "choices made individually through the marketplace are not inherently more sacrosanct than choices made collectively through the political process"—a fundamental point because frequently sloppy (or dishonest) thinkers claim that the ethical principle of respect for freedom of choice and personal rights *does* give some special preeminence to one form of choice over another. Such a claim deprives individuals of their democratic political rights, even as it proposes to entrench their economic rights. "One person, one vote" is subordinated to "one dollar, one vote." Nevertheless, a conflict remains between individual and collective choice processes, which goal 7 suppresses.

KD is well aware that this general collection of Good Things involves conflicts and necessitates trade-offs. But the specification of criteria to be applied to the evaluation of strategies, which might clarify the terms of this trade-off, in fact represents a shift away from emphasis on the goals themselves. They become just one collection of *desiderata*—pious hopes rather than hard targets—to be balanced against considerations of *realpolitik*.

Her proposed criteria for evaluating specific proposals are listed as

1. contribution to social goals (the seven listed above)
2. costs, including both total costs to society and distribution of costs between public and private budgets

3. acceptability to patients and providers
4. administrative feasibility
5. political feasibility

These criteria seem to be a blend of goals and constraints. Recall that cost-effectiveness of the health care system was originally a goal, yet now system costs emerge as a criterion. What's the difference? It may be that, as KD emphasized at the seminar, public and private dollars are not treated equally by the political system. A proposal that would significantly reduce the costs of health care to the United States as a whole (*e.g.*, as a percentage of Gross National Product), or moderate its increase, but that would at the same time transfer a larger proportion of those costs to the public (federal or state) budget—exactly what the Canadian public insurance systems have done—might run into heavy political opposition from those focusing on the public component of costs alone. But if so, surely that is a question of political feasibility, criterion 5? What is left of criterion 2 that is not included in either criterion 5 or goal 5?

The same question might be raised about criterion 3. Again, if free choice is a goal (7) and political and administrative feasibility are criteria or constraints, what is left for acceptability as a separate criterion? This is far from trivial because it would be hopelessly naive (which KD most assuredly is not) to imagine that *any* policy that promises to be effective in improving the efficiency of health care delivery, thereby lowering its rate of cost escalation, will be acceptable to providers. Since, by definition, health care costs *are* providers' incomes, in aggregate, a strict criterion of acceptability to providers must conflict with criterion 2 and defeat goal 5.

In practice, all significant changes in health care policy, in the United States or out of it, that have extended public insurance and/or public controls over the cost or content of medical practice have been bitterly opposed by the medical profession in particular. Sometimes they win; sometimes they lose; sometimes there are partial gains for both sides, and the net winners and losers may not be apparent for a number of years. But always there is a battle. The rhetoric of "acceptability" is simply part of the preliminary posturing by both sides trying to portray the other as in some sense the "aggressor." (For greater concreteness, consider how KD's recommendation of mandatory assignment will meet the acceptability criterion. More below.)

This discussion of goals versus criteria may appear to have an element of nit-picking to it, and to some extent it does. It suggests, however, that the logical structure of the KD paper is not nearly as tight as appears on the surface, and that the linkage from her broad, generally acceptable but conflicting and loosely specified goals to her policy proposals is rather more a matter of faith than of logic or argument. (Lest this seem unduly harsh, it is a disadvantage that most of us share. The Canadian public insurance system certainly redistributes the financial burdens of care in a way that most of us find more equitable than any private system; it almost certainly improves access, particularly for the poor and elderly, but it is hard indeed to find evidence that it results in improved general health status, KD's goals 1 and 2.) The criterion section of the paper seems to me to provide a sort of cover under which the scenery is changed, and we get down to specifics, heavily conditioned if not primarily determined by KD's judgments (no doubt well-informed, certainly more so than mine) about what is politically feasible in the present or future U.S. context and climate.

The concrete proposals of KD's paper are grouped under four heads, the first of which is clearly identified as the central set of proposals.

1. Extension of acute health care insurance coverage
2. Long-term care coverage through Medicare, including expanded home health benefits as well as nursing home care
3. System reform through promotion of the growth of HMOs, PPOs, and preventive and primary care
4. Provider payment reform, for both hospitals and physicians

The first set of proposals has a number of components, but in total it amounts to the development of universal health insurance coverage to at least minimum uniform benefit standards, albeit through a multiplicity of insurance carriers. It is a three-track system, or three-legged stool, built on Medicare, Medicaid, and mandatory employer coverage, but extended to cover the entire U.S. population.

All employers with twenty or more employees would be required to provide coverage for their full-time employees, spouses, and dependents. Deductibles and coinsurance would be permitted, but subject to an overall legal ceiling on annual out-of-pocket costs to patients. There would be specific requirements of choices of HMO and/or PPO coverage. The employer would be required to pay at least 75 percent of premium costs, with the stipulation that the federal government would pick up through a tax credit any costs (for the required minimum plan) beyond 5 percent of payroll. Persons leaving employment must be permitted to continue to buy coverage through the group, for themselves and their dependents, at group rates. (This seems to leave open a very important junction point with Medicare. Must retiring employees be permitted to continue in the employer plan, with Medicare as a secondary insurer? If yes, then the number of employer plans hitting the 5 percent ceiling will rise steadily over time.)

Medicare would be expanded to cover everyone over sixty-five (not already in a mandated employer plan), plus all the disabled, with the hospital and medical components merged and extended to the entire eligible population. Current premiums for supplementary medical care insurance would be replaced with an "income-related premium" with a ceiling and a floor that for a compulsory program would be another name for a tax. Ceilings would be placed on annual out-of-pocket payments; any outlays for an individual or family beyond these ceilings would be entirely reimbursed by Medicare. In addition, the government would market an optional Medi-gap policy to cover the present "cost-sharing" provisions of Medicare, with premiums set at actuarially fair levels.

Perhaps the most important changes for the longer run, and possibly the "Trojan Horse" of the whole proposal, is the feature that Medicaid "would be expanded to provide acute health care benefits to the entire population falling outside employer-mandated coverage and Medicare." Complete coverage would be provided to the poor, and everyone else could buy coverage in return for a sliding-scale, income-related premium. Such a proposal would go far to transfer Medicaid from its present status as a "charity" program through which "we" provide support for "them"—with all that that implies—to a "social insurance" program in which some beneficiaries, at least, have "earned" their entitlements.

But would the expanded Medicaid be compulsory or voluntary? A certain ambiguity surrounds this proposal because, if the total package is to be truly universal—covering the whole population—and if Medicaid is to be the "insurer of last resort," then it must be compulsory for everyone not covered by Medicare or an approved, mandated, employer plan. But the KD proposal does not actually say that it will be compulsory; rather, it refers to benefits "available to others not eligible" for other coverage. The political feasibility of *requiring* large numbers of people to join Medicaid and pay associated premiums may be questionable, but if this is not contemplated, then the claim of universality is hollow.

The Medicaid proposal may be a "Trojan Horse" because KD may in fact envision the progressive expansion of the "insurer of last resort" function. If the principle of universality can be established, helped along perhaps by rather generous ratios of benefits to premiums in the new "social insurance" form of Medicaid, then there might be a slow attrition of mandated employer plans into Medicaid. The growth of small business and part-time employment, if it continues, would increase Medicaid enrollment as well. And if such enrollment became respectable, no longer "charity," then employers who were hard pressed by the requirements of the mandated system and/or running up against the 5 percent of payroll limits might well seek to contract their employees into Medicaid.

Eventually, a respectable and largely premium-financed Medicaid might be merged with Medicare, and the nucleus of a national health insurance scheme would be in place.

If this is KD's vision, it is certainly not spelled out anywhere in so many words. But her proposal includes changes that represent important steps in that direction, though not identified as such. I would list these as

1. adoption of the principle of universal coverage, through Medicaid as insurer of last resort
2. shifting of funding sources either explicitly to general revenues or to "income-related" or "sliding-scale" premiums for benefit programs that are either compulsory or ambiguous as to enrollment
3. capping the out-of-pocket liabilities of patients, thus moving from ceilings to protect the insurance carrier to ceilings to protect the insured patient
4. moving toward standardization of minimum coverage, through both extended and improved Medicare and Medicaid benefits and mandated patterns of employer coverage

To me, this looks like easing in of universal, tax-financed national health insurance under other names and forms while trying to minimize resistance by a combination of maintaining or even expanding markets for private insurers (though not for Medi-gap insurers, where the load factors are presumably highest). The proposal involves a substantial extension of mandatory coverage, including Supplementary Medical Insurance (Part B) under Medicare and uniform employer-provided coverage, and a significant shift away from out-of-pocket payment (the caps on annual outlays) and toward tax finance (compulsory, "income-related premiums") related at least partially to ability to pay. KD's long-term care proposal is also rooted in these concepts, being financed by an "income-related premium" and "automatically" covering all those eligible for Medicare.

For political purposes, language is unquestionably of the essence. In substance, however, the KD proposal looks to me like a careful political calculation as to just how far one might be able to go toward tax-financed, universal, comprehensive coverage through a collection of separate but coordinated proposals with other names, each of which falls a bit short of the overall goal, and each of which will be phased in over time.

Relative to the present system, the KD proposal would be a substantial improvement. It would be more efficient and less costly to administer and much more equitable in financing and coverage. Many of the current irrationalities of Medicare, such as its peculiar split of hospital and physician coverage and its structure of deductibles and copayment that just create a large market for high-cost (in terms of load factors) private Medi-gap insurance, would be removed. Perhaps more important, the current situation imposes severe economic burdens on many of the sick elderly as well as on the rest of the population who have either no, or (often unknowingly) grossly inadequate insurance. The KD proposal caps the potential liabilities of Medicare beneficiaries, ensures basic protection for most employees and their dependents (including those on short-term unemployment), and provides an "insurer of last resort" for everyone else.

Relative to an overt national health insurance system, however, the proposal would be both less efficient and less equitable. It would be less efficient because the "three-legged stool" with one large leg of mandated and regulated employer-based coverage would still involve a large amount of administrative duplication and wasted motion and high overhead costs relative to a sole-source funding system. It would be less equitable because the various premium sources are still imperfectly related to ability to pay (although such general revenue sources as the income tax are also far from perfect either) and, principally, because despite the caps on individual out-of-pocket payments—which are an important step forward relative to the present situation—the KD proposal still involves a substantial element of "taxing the sick." It still augments the physical and emotional burdens of illness with the financial burdens of care, for which there is no equity case whatever.

But it may be that the incompleteness and residual inadequacies of the KD proposal are simply the price exacted by the inadequacies of the American political system—residual costs of the American Revolution—as it were. (That event is habitually regarded by Americans as some sort of triumph; it may be recalled that it was seen by a number of Canadians as a most unfortunate mistake.)

Interestingly, KD does *not* justify the retention of a significant component of out-of-pocket finance by the all too common arguments of economists that are echoed in the financial press. The superficial story is that direct charges to patients are necessary to prevent "frivolous" overuse of services and, thus, to control system costs. The evidence is quite otherwise. Out-of-pocket charges may influence decisions to seek care, particularly by lower-income individuals, but have no moderating influence on overall system costs. Internationally, greater reliance on direct charges is associated with *higher* costs, and the relationship is probably causal.

But KD's argument for retention is different and has two strands. First, the political reality is that public expenditure on health care is perceived as different from private expenditure. A plan that simply transfers costs from individual patients to the general public will be seen as a higher-cost plan and will thus encounter more political resistance. Moreover, so long as, misled by half-baked folk wisdom or equally half-baked economists, many people believe that out-of-pocket charges help to contain overall costs, a proposal will need to include such charges to appear "fiscally responsible."

Second, however, in the course of the seminar, KD suggested that the elimination of all direct charges to patients under the Medicare plan would not be the most appropriate use of scarce public funds. Since there are many other things that could be done with the same money that might have a more significant impact on health and well-being, elimination of out-of-pocket charges, once they have been capped, should not be a high priority.

This argument amounts to virtually overt acceptance of a tax on the sick, since it is formulated entirely in terms of the political difficulty of raising revenue for "good causes." Logically, it suggests that KD should be in favor of *raising* the cap on out-of-pocket payments under Medicare if she could be sure that the federal outlays thus saved would be channeled into, say, Alzheimer's clinics. Does an unjust tax become acceptable if the money it raises is well spent?

Underfunded or Overfunded

In fact KD's argument is perilously close at this point to that used by medical associations in Canada: "The health care system is 'underfunded,' because governments cannot or will not allocate enough resources (as judged by us) to health care. The solution is to raise the extra money by direct charges, preferably administered by individual physicians in the form of extra-billing—direct billing of patients at rates above the official fee schedules." KD would apparently disagree with this, since later in her paper she recommends mandatory assignment—no extra billing—but that presumably would only be because she would disagree with the Canadian physicians' definition of "underfunding" (*i.e.*, that they would like higher incomes). If the money could be used for some more meritorious purpose, she would presumably favor increased direct charges.

This is not only a rather peculiar argument about appropriate tax bases, it also implies rejection of the hypothesis of "flat of the curve medicine"—that in aggregate the U.S. health care system is if anything *overfunded*. Further increases in total spending will not lead to improvements in health outcomes—the benefit curve is flat. Resources should perhaps be reallocated, but not in total expanded, because in aggregate they are now being wasted on a large scale. This view is held by a number of observers, including Alain Enthoven and myself, and it leads us into the most serious shortcoming of the KD proposal and the greatest corresponding strength of the AE proposal.

The KD proposal is curiously old-fashioned in its principal thrust. (One might even call it a CHIP off the old block.) It has four sections—two dealing with the extension of benefits and two with the reform of the delivery system and of the payment process. But it is the extension of acute health care insurance coverage that really forms the heart of the proposal and engages the author's principal attention. From reading Davis's proposal, one would never guess that cost containment and, in more sophisticated quarters, value for money had been for a number of years at or near the top of the health-policy agenda. How does one prevent the health care system from absorbing larger and larger shares of the nation's income?

A proposal that sidesteps that issue almost completely seems to me to be open to obvious and strong political attack. If the United States is unable to contain its medical-care cost explosion at present or to assure that its citizens receive benefits at all commensurate with the resources they give up, how much worse will the problem be under the extended system that KD proposes?

Cost Containment

KD has three sorts of responses, representing quite different approaches, which are articulated with each other only in the sketchiest way. First, the KD proposal would encourage the growth of alternatives to fee-for-service practice. All three of the legs on her insurance stool would be required to offer enrollees a choice of one or more federally qualified HMOs and/or PPOs, depending on availability. Second, she would provide increased funding for particular diseases such as Alzheimer's, and for preventive and primary care. Third, she would modify the payment process for both hospitals and physicians. Yet in fact, none of these represent any significant response to the problem of cost containment and system management.

On the first point, it is well known that HMOs can significantly reduce rates of hospital utilization and, as a result, lower costs of care for their beneficiary populations. But there is not yet any evidence that such organizations lower the total costs of care in the regions in which they operate, even in areas of high penetration such as Minneapolis or Hawaii. Nor is it clear whether they flatten the trend of cost escalation or simply follow it at a slightly lower level. As AE emphasizes, the efficiency benefits of HMOs, PPOs, and alternative delivery systems generally can emerge only in the context of a genuinely competitive market, which has not been present up to now in the United States; and there is nothing in the KD proposal that would move any farther down that road. Indeed, in the course of the seminar, KD expressed her belief that in spite of the very rapid growth of HMOs and PPOs, their enrollments were still so small, and would be for the foreseeable future, that they would not be a significant feature of the policy landscape.

From reading Davis's proposal, one would never guess that cost containment and, in more sophisticated quarters, value for money had been for a number of years at or near the top of the health-policy agenda. How does one prevent the health care system from absorbing larger and larger shares of the nation's income?

On the second point, it has been a popular misconception, widely promoted by politicians, that preventive services have the capacity to reduce health care need, and thereby utilization, and thereby costs. For some this is an argument for developing an alternative "preventive" care system; for others it is an excuse for victim-blaming ("illness is all the patient's own fault") and for reducing public support; and for still others the preventive care concept is a dream of relief from the pressures of funding an ever-growing system. The hard facts are that there is no evidence that preventive care, however meritorious in itself, will lead to the "withering away" of the curative system and thus provide a solution to the problems of cost containment and efficient management. An apple a day will not make the doctor's bill go away. Indeed, to the extent that it is successful, preventive care may very well, by extending life, *increase* costs. But that it another story.

KD does not of course claim that prevention is a solution to the cost-control problem, but her juxtaposition of recommendations leaves this interpretation open. In any case, it is not a solution, and we are left then with her proposals for reimbursement reform.

Here we have two proposals—fine tuning and extension of the prospective payment system for hospitals (DRGs) and a binding fee schedule for physicians. These proposals deserve serious consideration, because as the Canadian experience makes clear, tight control of the payment process *can* both contain cost escalation and provide some degree of indirect stimulus to improved system efficiency. Unfortunately, I do not believe that the proposals sketched in so lightly in the KD paper would in fact provide this control.

It is true that the Medicare prospective payment system for hospitals, introduced in October of 1983, has markedly reduced the rate of cost escalation in U.S. hospitals, through 1985 at least. This has come about through a substantial drop in average lengths of stay per acute hospital episode. It has also been associated with tighter preadmission screening—resulting in a fall in admission rates—and increased efforts by private insurers, such that utilization has fallen among the under-sixty-five population as well. KD's recommendations to encourage states to extend the system to all payers might extend these savings as well.

But the current record suggests that the effects of the PPS/DRG system have been almost entirely on admissions; it has not touched the underlying trends in cost escalation per patient day or intensity of servicing. If so, then its effects will be "one shot," persisting only so long as lengths of stay keep falling. They cannot fall indefinitely and may already be near a lower bound. Moreover, there is reason to believe that some of the "savings" in the hospital sector may be showing up as increased costs in the physicians' services, in the nursing home, and particularly in the insurance overhead sectors. The rise in the costs of prepayment, administration, and management in the overall U.S. system from 1983 to 1985 almost exactly match the reduction in hospital costs (relative to trend) that may be the result of PPS/DRGs.

Finally, the "fine tuning" that KD proposes (my word, not hers) includes "adjusting the DRG payment rate for teaching hospitals to take into account the complexity of cases treated." While unassailable in principle, in practice all suggested methods of such adjustment that I am aware of open the door to the institution's manipulating the categorization of the patient by its labeling decision to increase its own revenue. The "adjustment" thus undercuts the whole point of the PPS, which is to separate the hospital's revenue per patient from its own treatment decisions. No solution to this dilemma is proposed.

In sum, then, I must conclude that KD's proposals for hospital-funding reform do not promise any significant advance on the problems of either cost escalation or treatment efficiency. The proposals of the Harvard Medicare Project, for development of state-based all-payer global budgets, seem to me a good deal more promising for cost control in the context of a regulatory system.

Fee Control

As for fee control, here the Canadian experience has quite clearly shown that this is an effective method for limiting the escalation of medical costs. In the United States, physicians' fees have quite consistently outrun the general inflation rate for at least the last four decades. In Canada, they did so prior to the introduction of the universal public insurance plans; since then they have run at or behind the inflation rate.

But the Canadian experience also shows, as does U.S. experience with "fee freezes," that physicians have a great deal of scope for manipulating their billing patterns to expand their total receipts even though charges for individual items remain constant. Containing this requires an ongoing and quite sophisticated negotiating process—a "managed" fee schedule—not a one-time decision combined with a mechanical escalation rule. The reimbursing agency must take an interest in, and negotiate, the structure of the schedule, the rules governing payment and interpretation, and the rates for individual items—or it will lose its (or more accurately the taxpayer's) shirt. None of these considerations—who is to do the negotiating, how, with whom, or even any recognition that the process is of the essence—are included in the KD proposal.

Indeed KD describes her proposal as "revenue-neutral," implying that it is *not* intended as a way of limiting physician receipts or insurance outlays. It may be that this revenue-neutrality refers only to the first year after introduction, since the pegging of the schedule to the Consumer Price Index implies a reduction of 1 to 2 percent in the annual rate of increase of U.S. physicians' fees—in the past they have always outrun the CPI. (If the schedule is not very carefully designed to prevent it, however, "fee creep" can easily eat up 2 percent a year, and a lot more besides.)

But the introduction process is ambiguous as well. If a uniform schedule is adopted, in the first year some physicians will be above it, and some will be below. If those above it are not to have their fees reduced but only frozen until inflation raises the overall schedule to their level, then revenue-neutrality would require that those below not be raised to the schedule, but merely held at *their* previous levels. You cannot raise those below to the average, hold others above the average, and still be revenue neutral! You could, of course, use the whole of the increase in the second year to raise those at the low end, thus giving them more than CPI until they caught up with the schedule, but that is not spelled out. One is left with the impression that this section is rather an afterthought.

The imposition of mandatory assignment is a right and proper part of any approach to fixed-fee-schedule reimbursement, particularly if it is proposed that certain physicians will be "equalized down" either immediately or over time. It is also essential to ensure that services are available to insured beneficiaries. But the proposal refers in this section only to Medicare. Presumably the fee schedule will also be binding on Medicaid, and on the mandated employer plans as well. This might be a powerful marketing tool for employers, though hard to articulate with the growth of PPOs. It will, however, be political dynamite among physicians, requiring careful constituency building in support.

But the discussion of physicians' reimbursement totally ignores one of the principal problems for any system of universal coverage and fixed-fee reimbursement—the surplus of physicians. The supply of physicians in the United States is currently growing about 2 percent per year faster than the population and will, in the absence of major intervention, continue to do so for decades. At present, per capita utilization of physicians' services is rising at about the same rate as physician supply; some say this is simply coincidence, but most see a causal connection. The connection will not be weakened by any of KD's proposals.

The physician surplus builds a permanent cost-inflation factor into the health care system, in both the corresponding expansion of utilization and costs of physicians' services and the pressure to specialize and subspecialize to survive in a crowded market. The latter process generates further demand for more and more technologically sophisticated hospital and clinic interventions and the specialized auxiliary personnel to support them—driven not so much by the health needs of patients as by the economic needs of ever more physicians. The impact of this expanding surplus on overall costs can only be offset by reducing physicians' average incomes (as the AE proposal intends, inter alia, to do) or by putting some other group out of their jobs (such as hospital nurses). It is intimately linked with the process of physician reimbursement, yet does not enter KD's consideration at all.

Political Feasibility

The KD proposal seems to me to be the most carefully worked out in terms of its political "saleability"; it is packaged (in many small bundles) and labeled so as to allay suspicion, is based on careful cost calculations of the sort that would be most acceptable to Congress and the budget office, and is characterized at almost every point by a willingness to settle for half or three-quarters of a loaf. It reflects its author's long experience with Washington. I have considerable unease about the political response to some of its components: (a) How will employers react to mandatory health insurance, and can that be sold? (b) Mandatory physician assignment is essential, but can it be done? I am not sure if all of this has been thought through, but KD's experience in such matters is greater than mine.

What is clear to me is that if such a program could be achieved, it would be, as noted above, a very long step forward in both access to care and equity of funding and a partial step toward reducing the inefficiency of the insurance process itself—the overhead costs of the present U.S. system.

But the great gap in the proposal, which I believe would be fatal to its chances of adoption—and if it were adopted would certainly lead to its very rapid modification—is that it does not in any serious way address the issues of cost control and efficiency. The evidence is, I believe, overwhelming that the present system of health care in the United States is incapable of setting any upper limit on its resource demands. Such limits must either be imposed from outside, as the Canadian system does, or else the U.S. system has to be restructured so that it is capable of reaching an internal balance, as the AE proposal is intended to achieve.

Moreover, the evidence is equally compelling that the present U.S. acute-care system is arbitrary and wasteful in the way it uses the resources it absorbs from other social uses, that it does a bad job of supplying value for money, and that it lacks internal incentives or "adaptive intelligence" for learning from or improving this situation. Cost escalation would not be a problem if we believed that the U.S. health care system were yielding commensurate benefits. The extensive evidence accumulating all over the United States for decades of costly interventions that are arbitrarily applied and unevaluated and that employ overtrained and overpaid personnel says that it is not

Long-Term Care

Nor is this an issue only in the acute-care system. The present U.S. long-term care system comes in for much criticism—which sounds to me justified—for its excessive focus on support associated with medical and nursing care. But the motivation, I think, is understandable, even if the means are inappropriate. The restrictions are intended to place some limit on the numbers of people in long-term care and on the costs in an area where needs are much more difficult to define than in acute care (and those are difficult enough). The alternative, however, is some sort of regionally based assessment system by panels of professionals with budgets who are responsible for determining who is admitted, to what form of care, and for how long.

Robert and Rosalie Kane have described and analyzed several variants of this approach in some of the Canadian provinces, and they approve it; but whether or not one accepts this particular approach, it is inescapable that any long-term care system with any pretensions to adequacy *must* have some form of system gatekeeper. Equally obviously, the practicing physician has neither the training to perform this role, nor is his or her primary responsibility to the patient consistent with it. Yet KD's proposals on long-term care, however meritorious in general terms, are totally silent on this critical point. It is left to RK to wrestle with.

System Management and Cost Control

In the 1960s, these problems of system management and cost control were not so apparent, and an essentially "pay the bills" program such as KD proposes—of attaching more people more closely to the existing delivery system—was the dominant approach to health insurance in the United States and elsewhere. In the 1980s, it is curiously old-fashioned. Yet one wonders. Karen Davis knows all this. She might quite legitimately argue that, since the problems of cost escalation and inefficiency in health care are so acute in the present incomplete and fragmented U.S. system, there is no reason to assume that they would be any worse in the fairer system she proposes. She is not trying to solve all the problems, only those of the many vulnerable people inadequately served by, or left entirely out of, the present system. And that is enough of a challenge.

She may even, covertly, be quite aware that her proposals would bring the problems of system regulation or reform out to front and center, necessitating a serious attempt at solution. By saddling government with a still larger share of the growing total of expenditure, her plan might rebalance the political forces and create a stronger constituency for cost control and system reform. It should be noted that her plan puts the federal government very heavily at risk for the *marginal* dollar of expenditure. Once the liabilities of patients are capped, and to the extent that employer plans run up against the 5 percent of payroll ceiling, further expenditure increases come dollar for dollar out of public revenues. The current U.S. pattern of "cost-pass-through," whereby every participant in the health care funding process tries to shift costs to someone else rather than accepting the burden of managing them, would be largely ended. Conceivably this could be the most significant part of the proposal.

But if such is the intent, it is well hidden in the paper, and no hint is given as to the need for or the nature of this process of controlling and managing the delivery system itself. And I cannot help but feel that as the share of the U.S. national income devoted to health care seems inexorably to increase, it is both understandable and perhaps appropriate that health policy should become increasingly driven by budgetary policy. A proposal that does not speak to the management issues, but instead seeks to widen access to a system that seems unable to achieve long-run cost stability (and whose days may therefore be numbered) may have difficulty gathering a constituency.

THE ENTHOVEN SYSTEM

Alain Enthoven's proposals, on the other hand, are virtually the inverse of KD's—looking forward where hers look backward, strong where hers are weak, and weak where hers are strong. It is worth emphasizing again, however, the fundamental agreement in underlying philosophy that is also shared by RK and myself and that AE makes very clear at the beginning: the need for a universal and comprehensive insurance system, with no one denied access to care on the grounds of inability to pay or subjected to extreme financial hardship as a result of illness. (The word "extreme," which AE uses here, may leave room for some negotiation, but it is probably not critical.) In the process, however, AE would bring about a revolutionary transformation of the delivery system for health care in the United States.

There are four principal "players" in the AE system: patients, providers, sponsors, and government (although particular government agencies may also play the role of sponsors for some populations). The concrete model for their interaction is the current health insurance system offered by Stanford University to its employees, in which the university plays the role of sponsor, but the Federal Employees' Health Benefits Plan (FEHBP) is another large and long-established example of a sponsoring organization.

In this framework, each individual or family is enrolled with a sponsoring organization, which offers the enrollee a choice (open to periodic revision) among a restricted set of health service plans. Providers are organized into Competitive Medical Plans (CMPs), each offering a package of services, terms, conditions, and costs. The enrollee signs up with a particular CMP for a period of time—say a year—and that CMP agrees to provide comprehensive care to that enrollee for that period in return for a preset capitation payment (subject, perhaps, to particular forms of additional payments for specific services, determined in advance).

Traditional fee-for-service medicine, with the patient having unrestricted choice of physician and the physician having unrestricted choice of therapy and of fee setting, could be thought of as a sort of "residual" CMP (although in practice not a very competitive one) in which the payments received by the "organization"—the collectivity of physicians and hospitals that the patient might consult—are not fixed in advance but are proportionate to the services provided.

The capitation-reimbursed CMP would be under two powerful sets of incentives. On the one hand, it must strive to hold down the costs of providing care to its consumer/patients because its revenues are determined in advance by the capitation amount. Too much servicing, too high incomes to its personnel, or just plain inefficient management will lead to losses and possible bankruptcy. On the other hand, poor service to its clientele—long waits for appointments, surly or obviously incompetent staff, poor facilities—will lead to enrollees leaving the CMP at the next enrollment period and, thus, to complete loss of the capitation revenue. Attempts to pass cost increases along to enrollees in the form of higher capitation rates will bring similar results. Thus, the CMP is motivated to be efficient by internal economic pressures, backed up by competition among CMPs for the capitation business itself.

Sponsors—Regulation and Evaluation

In this process, however, the sponsor plays a critical role. It is notorious that patients are not sufficiently informed or otherwise equipped to negotiate on even terms with providers of care; this disadvantage will be magnified as providers become organized into multiphysician groups, integrated with hospitals, and tied directly to a payment organization. Patients may be able to detect poor servicing that takes the form of long waits, dirty or broken facilities, and surly staff, but poor quality medicine can kill a great many patients who die in perfect confidence that they have received the best of care. That, after all, is the fundamental rationale for public regulation of physicians and other professionals.

The AE system envisions a continuation of present forms of professional regulation, though with some modification to prevent them from being used, as they commonly are, as economic weapons to suppress competition and innovation and thus to exploit patients. But the sponsoring organization will also be collecting data on the comparative performance of CMPs, both within and outside the "portfolio" of choices that it offers to its registrants. Sponsors may pool their efforts in this regard, to develop the large databases that AE emphasizes are necessary for effective evaluation of delivery organizations.

As part of this process, the sponsor will also be a natural client for clinical epidemiology, or evaluative research more generally, on the sorts of medical interventions that are effective and on the efficient ways of providing them. And CMPs will be equally motivated to develop and use this information, so long as they are in competition with each other for enrollees, because the CMP that identifies an inappropriate or ineffective form of servicing can discontinue it, thereby lowering its costs and either increasing its profits (or if nonprofit, its surplus revenues for other purposes) or lowering the capitation rate it charges in order to promote increased enrollment. The CMP that lags behind, providing ineffective services, will lose money, or patients, or both.

The sponsor thus has responsibility for maintaining competition among the CMPs it offers to its members and preventing them from colluding in either pricing or choice of technique; it can add or drop CMPs from its approved list. It therefore has much more influence on this market than any one individual could ever hope to have.

The sponsor also manages the payment process. If the sponsor is an employer, it would deduct employee contributions from their paychecks, add its own share of contributions, and forward these to the CMP the employee has chosen from the list made available by the sponsor. Capitation payments need not, however, be uniform; CMPs might offer different plans at different prices, and employees might choose a high-cost, high-benefit plan or a low-cost, low-benefit one. Moreover, the employer might—probably would—define its contribution in flat-rate terms rather than as a proportion of the annual rate charged by the CMP so that employees choosing low-cost plans would have a higher proportion of their total premiums paid by the employer. This is intended to transmit further pressure through to the CMPs to contain costs. If the employer pays a flat contribution, then every dollar by which the capitation rate of a CMP exceeds that of its competitors is a dollar out of the pockets of each of its enrollees.

To reinforce the competitive pressure, the AE plan would also remove the tax deductibility of employer-paid health insurance premiums and make them taxable in the hands of the employee (as currently applies in Canada in those provinces that still finance part of their public hospital and medical care plans through premiums, but does not apply to private dental or extended health benefit coverage). There would then be no advantage for employees in trying to bargain with the employer to pick up a larger share of the capitation fee; such a benefit would be taxable just as if it were wages. Again, the employee is being required to bear the costs of his/her decisions among alternative CMPs and, thus, the pressure is maintained on CMPs to control costs.

The proposal to remove the tax deductibility of employer-paid premiums has two further advantages that AE emphasizes. It removes a tax concession that is blatantly regressive in being of much greater value to taxpayers in the highest tax brackets and providing a substantial amount of new revenue that could be contributed by government to help fund the reformed health care system. It has the disadvantage, however, that it seems to be intensely unpopular with everyone except economists.

Sponsors would quite quickly realize, however, the advantages of offering a portfolio of less expensive CMPs, by restricting the benefit package, as well as the disadvantages of acting on behalf of individuals with chronic or otherwise expensive conditions. Thus, government regulators have a critical role in creating and maintaining a regulatory environment in which competition serves to promote efficiency, not just to drop people with the greatest problems and/or to degrade the quality of the insurance "product." In principle, informed "consumers" might monitor the sponsor's offering, but enrollees generally are very sketchily informed about the contents of their insurance contracts until it is too late. That is why the AE plan has sponsors, and the plan does not envision a competitive market in sponsors, only in CMPs. Sponsors do not compete, they manage the competition among CMPs, so if their performance is to be controlled, it must be through public regulation.

The proposal to remove the tax deductibility of employer-paid premiums . . . removes a tax concession that is blatantly regressive . . . and it provides a substantial amount of new revenue that could be contributed by government to help fund the reformed health care system. It has the disadvantage, however, that it seems to be intensely unpopular with everyone except economists.

In the AE plan, it is. Government sets the contents of the basic comprehensive plan that must be offered by all CMPs in the sponsor's stable and the terms of enrollment and coverage for the people for whom the sponsor is responsible. Government also continues the regulation of providers, separate from the payment process. And it might well manage or contract for the process of evaluation of the effectiveness of different forms of care, both to support the efforts of sponsors individually or collectively and to target sponsors who were making no such effort.

Increased Efficiency

The fundamental idea—the driving force—of the AE plan is the improvement of the efficiency of the U.S. health care system, precisely the idea that is virtually absent from the KD proposal. It presupposes, therefore, that there is a very high level of waste and misapplied effort in the present system, so that intensified pressures on providers to cut costs will not lead to reduced quality and increased morbidity and mortality. AE emphasizes that it is *poor* quality medicine that is expensive medicine because it leads to further problems. There are numerous examples of the validity of this principle, such as small hospitals doing complex surgical procedures infrequently, with higher cost and poorer outcomes, or underutilized surgeons with similar effects. Excessive or duplicative diagnostic work, without any clear strategy of investigation, can also lead to unnecessary interventions as well as higher costs. And so on.

On the other hand, it remains true that the cheapest form of intervention is to do nothing at all, now or ever, and just to let nature take its course, and this does not yield the best results. I find the evidence as convincing as does AE that the savings are there to be made and that pressures to contain costs need not lead to a deterioration of system outcomes. That is, after all, a principal message of the Canadian experience. The critical question is, will the institutional framework that AE proposes focus these competitive pressures to promote greater efficiency while still maintaining a universal and comprehensive system of insurance coverage with the economic burdens equitably distributed across the population?

I find the AE proposal somewhat unclear and incomplete on the process whereby the whole population is to be linked into the competitive system, and what their cost burdens are going to be—precisely the descriptive points on which the KD proposal was strongest. The problems seem to me to fall under two major heads: (1) creation and motivation of a system of sponsors to cover the whole population, and (2) adapting the financing system to allow for the variance in population risk status. It may be more convenient to discuss these in reverse order.

Enrollee Risk Status

The AE proposal applies most naturally to a group of enrollees who are more or less identical in their probability of suffering illness or injury over the next year. From the point of view of a sponsor, or a CMP, they are indistinguishable, and the same capitation rate would apply to each. Some will actually experience illness and use care, others will not. So the actual expenditure will differ across individuals, but will average out for a large group. If some people choose more expensive CMPs because they are more convenient, or have thicker carpets, or offer services above the guaranteed basic comprehensive package—cosmetic surgery, for example, or dental care—there is no reason in justice or economic efficiency why they should not pay full rate for these, without subsidy from the employer or the taxpayer. If they choose higher-cost CMPs that are simply inefficient or overly generous to their physicians or employees, a fortiori, we do not want others to subsidize their choices. The whole point of the AE proposal is to get the high-cost providers to clean up their act.

But people *do* differ in their risk status or expectation of illness, not just in their actual experience. A CMP will quite properly want to be paid a higher capitation rate for older enrollees or for those who have chronic conditions. If it is not paid a capitation rate that corresponds to the higher risk of expense, the CMP will obviously be forced, by competitive pressures, to avoid enrolling such people. But if the capitation rate varies by risk category, can the sponsor's contribution remain constant? The arguments for placing the burden of differential costs on the individual— by making the sponsor's contribution a flat one and by making employer-paid benefits taxable—now work backwards; they subject people in the highest risk categories to the highest share of the capitation rate.

Even if the sponsor makes a contribution that varies with some index of the enrollee's risk status—say age and sex, as obvious though very incomplete examples—the employee's share will still amount to a larger payment for those who are in higher risk categories. Someone has to carry the burden of differential risk. If the CMP is required by regulation to carry it, there will be access problems for higher-risk people. If the CMP is (somehow) appropriately compensated, then the sponsor and the enrollee will have to share the extra cost. To the extent that sponsors limit their contributions to a flat amount per enrollee, the individual is exposed to an unjust distribution of burden. In concrete terms, older workers will have to pay more for their coverage than younger workers. But if sponsors pick up a larger share of the costs for higher-risk enrollees, then they have an obvious incentive to try to avoid enrolling high-risk individuals.

Does the government come to the rescue? In the AE plan, the federal government will make a payment to each individual or family of roughly 40 percent of the premium costs of their plan. This payment presumably goes to the sponsor and is proportionate to the total premium cost, regardless of how it is split between sponsor and enrollee. Also, although AE does not say so, I presume that if the sponsor discriminates among enrollees in setting premiums, each individual receives a federal subsidy proportionate to his or her *actual* premium, not the group average.

But government's role does not end there. It will also serve as sponsor for the Medicare population, for whom it will presumably pick up the share of costs that an employer otherwise would. In addition, state governments will presumably act as sponsors for Medicaid eligibles for whom they might add further supplementation. The federal subsidy to private plan premiums, however, deserves more attention in the context of the new AE plan. He suggests that it be proportional to plan premiums, up to a ceiling. On what other factors might the federal contribution to private plans be made conditional?

The answer at one extreme—none—seems clearly untenable. A flat federal payment to each sponsoring organization per person covered is clearly at odds with the realities of the differentials in disease, utilization, and cost incidence. The federal contribution will have to be related to some index based on personal characteristics and, almost certainly, on residence characteristics as well, to reflect regional differences in cost patterns. But once one goes beyond age, sex, and residence, the problems of identifying and monitoring risk status become extreme. Groups of people can be experience-rated, but payments on behalf of individuals are much more difficult to determine. What status categories should matter and by how much, and which individuals fall into those categories?

One can envision a very large book, a "Domesday Book," tabulating the different federal payments to be made on behalf of different types of individuals—and a good deal of conflict and litigation on the subject, which with changing technology and epidemiology need never settle down. As a concrete example, should larger payments be made to sponsors on behalf of homosexuals because of their higher risk of contracting AIDS?

Moreover, reliance on easy indicators like age is undermined by increasing evidence that the increase in health care costs with age is closely linked with terminal care and increased probability of high-cost chronic illness. For the majority of the aged who are healthy, health care costs are not much more than for the rest of the population.

Insofar as the federal payment fails to reflect the risk status of an individual or group, there is an economic incentive for a sponsoring organization to try to avoid (or encourage) enrollment of that individual— and an incentive for other members of the sponsor's population to cooperate in this discrimination. But even if the federal payment could be made proportionate to risk status, it still covers only about 40 percent of the total cost. The remaining 60 percent must still be partitioned among sponsor, individual, and CMP—and we assumed for the moment that the CMP bears none of it because capitation risks reflect risk status accurately. (The CMP, as provider of care, will usually have the best information available on an individual's actual risk status, since that arises in the course of health care utilization.) The same problems then arise of the dilemma between placing the burden of risk status on the individual, who may not be able to afford it (that is why private insurance breaks down for the people with greatest needs—an old and well-known story), or on the sponsor, which creates the incentive for the sponsor to select beneficiaries and avoid people of high risk.

Yet a third alternative would be for the federal government to pay 40 percent on average, but to pay a higher percentage for those in higher risk categories so as to try to equalize the absolute amount of the sponsor's and the individual's payment across risk categories. This might ameliorate the problems at the sponsor level, but it would lead to very much higher variance in federal payments, since they would not only respond to risk status but be highly leveraged by the implicit flat 60 percent share. The political and legal problems of compiling the "Domesday Book" would be an order of magnitude more difficult, as the financial consequences of epidemiological uncertainty would be much more severe.

(In fact AE's proposal goes in exactly the opposite direction, by placing an absolute cap on federal contributions. In consequence, people with higher premiums will receive a lower proportionate federal subsidy. This is perfectly logical as a way of encouraging cost consciousness in individual selection of plans, but it clearly penalizes any person or group whose higher premium is a reflection of higher risk status. The defensibility of this ceiling then turns on whether variance in premiums across different plans is primarily a function of provider behavior or of patient characteristics.)

Faced with this collection of undesirable alternatives, one is led to suspect that the bureaucratic mind would respond, understandably, with something as defensible as age, sex, and regional adjustment, with perhaps a few unambiguous conditions thrown in. Moreover, it is possible that the consequences of this approach might not be so serious, given that the elderly, disabled, and poor would already be included in publicly sponsored systems that had no incentive, or at least opportunity, to discriminate against them. For the employed population and their dependents, the variance of utilization experience and risk status may not be as serious a problem.

Indeed, some such judgment is implicit in AE's proposal that the federal payment be proportionate to plan premiums; he is implicitly assuming that, up to the ceiling, intergroup differences in average enrollee characteristics will be reflected in the premium, and intragroup differences will not be large enough to make premium or other forms of discrimination worthwhile. Perhaps so; after all, present provider-sponsored plans function with a much less logical and more inequitable form of federal subsidy through the tax system, as AE points out.

On the other hand, until recently, employees have not had the costs of benefits for individual employees spelled out for them. A system of capitation reimbursement to CMPs that will have to be differentiated by employee characteristics will place an explicit price tag on each employee and family, readily interpretable by the dimmest personnel manager and transmitted directly to the famous bottom line. The incentives to transfer the cost of high risk status to the employee through, say, a flat employer contribution to the premium or to transfer the employee through, say, "dehiring" are equally apparent.

Enthoven's Sponsors

That, however, leads into the other question raised above. Who are the sponsors, how are they motivated, and how do they acquire their enrollees? AE asserts that consumers play the most important role in his plan, but I believe the key role is that of the sponsors, and it is by no means clear to me that they are up to it. To illustrate, consider AE's archetypical sponsor, Stanford University. As an employer, it is

1. large, with a large pool of employees/risks
2. prosperous, with a stable and predictable revenue
3. nonprofit, or at least not-for-profit
4. responsible for a generally healthy population
5. an employer of people for whom there are few readily available close substitutes

This last point may be of some significance. Stanford, for example, employs Alain Enthoven and presumably values his services highly. If he were to die or suffer severe impairment of function, Stanford University would suffer a loss in terms of its reputation and perceived mission. He would not be easily or immediately replaceable, because the market in Alain Enthovens is at present quite thin. It is therefore prudential, as well as humane, for Stanford to take an interest in his well-being. The same would be true of a highly skilled member of a for-profit corporation—IBM, say, or GM.

Moreover, Stanford has the resources, both in finances and, most important, in management expertise, to do so. If they need epidemiological or economic advice, they know where to get the best available and how to use it.

"Enlightened" employers, who take an interest in the continued well-being of their employees, do so for good, sound business reasons. We may therefore expect that as a sponsor, Stanford, as well as IBM or GM, would put a considerable amount of effort and corporate resources into managing the care that their employees receive and would be penny-wise but pound-foolish to deal with a "cut-rate," low-quality CMP, saving money at the expense of the employees' health.

Consider, at the other end of the scale, a small business with few employees, high turnover, and many part-timers, operating on a shoestring in terms of both management and profits. For this firm, which may not have had an employee health plan at all, the AE plan involves a sort of triple step forward—mandated coverage extended to *all* employees, not just the full-timers, and involving not just the traditional premium-collecting and record-keeping functions but state-of-the-art management of a very complex health care system. And the incentives to do so are not there. One employee is very much like another, and if one becomes ill, or even dies (or less dramatically becomes fed up with the quality of care offered), there are plenty of fish in the sea. It is not like replacing AE!

Moreover, even under optimal conditions, one employee who develops an expensive illness might break the organization. In such circumstances, the employer/sponsor will have no choice but to be very selective in hiring, whatever the regulations say, and will have an obvious incentive to collude with the members of the approved list of CMPs for its employees to avoid high-cost interventions, even at some risk to employee health. This need not be outright refusal to provide certain interventions in any circumstances; extreme parsimony in application would do just as well. Nor need it be explicit. As someone has said about contract-funded academic research, "the milkman's horse does not need to be told where to stop."

Indeed, providing a choice among cut-rate CMPs may do the selection job automatically; the people most likely to experience unsatisfactory care and to be motivated to leave the employer as a result will, on average, be the people with health problems. The more fit or fortunate will not use the health care system much, if at all, and will not know of its quality.

Perhaps some form of multiemployer trust or reinsurance system can deal with the problems of scale economies in information assembly and risk bearing, and of learning by doing; but then, in effect, the umbrella organization becomes the sponsor—at one remove from the employees—and the relationship between employer and sponsor becomes problematic. Nor does the problem of conflict of interest between sponsor and employee disappear; it simply acquires an extra dimension.

The core of the difficulty is that when people have vulnerable interests that they are unable to protect for themselves, as they have when they confront the health care system, someone else must serve as their agent(s) in managing the transactions on their behalf and protecting their interests. Traditionally, physicians and, to a lesser extent, other professionals have done this; they serve as "sponsors" as well as providers. In the traditional form of national health insurance as extended by KD, physicians continue to act as sponsors.

How does one find sponsors for the self-employed, the part-timers, the employees of small business, the people who have no special characteristics that make them stand out of the labor pool and whose employers' financial and management resources are sufficiently stretched by the needs of daily survival (or in some cases, the demands of exceptional cupidity)? And if one can find such sponsors, what motivates them? . . . The problem of policing performance is likely to be severe.

AE's point is that in this conflict of interest between the sponsor and the provider roles, providers have served their own interests at least as well as those of their patients. The resulting system of care is wasteful of resources, unfair, in many respects ineffective or even unnecessarily harmful in the patterns of care it provides, and, over time, incapable of placing any limit on its economic demands on the rest of society. I believe the evidence supports him, and this is the telling criticism of KD's approach.

But the sponsors that AE proposes also suffer from a conflict of interest, though the patterns of interest are different. His Stanford University example, I believe, minimizes these conflicts and their potential costs and represents a best case, not a typical, much less a worst case, employer/sponsor. How does one find sponsors for the self-employed, the part-timers, the employees of small business, the people who have no special characteristics that make them stand out of the labor pool and whose employers' financial and management resources are sufficiently stretched by the needs of daily survival (or in some cases, the demands of exceptional cupidity)? And if one *can* find such sponsors, what motivates them? AE is rightly suspicious of broker/sponsors acting for a profit— there is too much opportunity for abuse of the conflict-of-interest situation. But if the role is simply assigned, the problem of policing performance is likely to be severe.

AE's response to this seems to me the right one. States (or perhaps lower-level geographic units) would serve as "sponsors of last resort," required to enroll anyone who is not part of some other sponsored plan—looking very much like KD's version of Medicaid. This emphasizes yet again that if one is serious about universality, one must either replace the current system with a truly universal one (as Canada did) or create an organization (or redefine an existing one) in which membership is compulsory for anyone *not* enrolled in some approved alternative. The control of quality in the range of CMPs offered by this residual sponsor and the balance of costs between enrollees (compulsory premiums) and the state (general revenues), which would be analogous to the issues settled by collective bargaining with private employers, would be settled through the political process.

Over time, however, it seems to me that the long-run dynamics will probably lead either to the state-based system's expanding its scope (smaller employers fold their people into it) or to convergence of characteristics of all systems to a de facto single system, with a rather peculiar and awkward administrative structure. (Is Germany not going this way?) Alternatively, one could imagine the state-based residual system becoming increasingly inferior in terms of either perceived quality and benefits or the distribution of cost burdens, such that universality would become progressively less and less meaningful. But I think it would be a very delicate balancing act indeed, to maintain the balance of advantages between the private and the residual public sponsoring systems such that neither dominated the other, and yet each remained different.

At the very least, I would expect the Medicare, Medicaid, and residual state sponsors to become very similar, if not consolidated, and to become larger as the population ages and the aged continue to increase their relative use of care faster than the rest of the population. Among the working population, shifts to more part-time and small-scale employment will also encourage the growth of the state insurer of last resort. Why go to the trouble of forming (and policing) a Multi-Employer Trust when one can just fold one's employees into the state system? But as the public system becomes larger, how can it avoid contracting with any given CMP? As the buyer becomes larger, its decisions spell survival or dissolution for potential contractors, and AE's correct characterization of the political process comes into play. The state has a difficult time, politically, if it is seen to wipe out an economic interest.

I would not wish to imply that AE has not thought about these issues or that he does not have answers to some of them in his paper for the AARP meeting and in other publications. And I am sensitive to his charge that an economist is someone who sees something working in practice and wonders if it will work in theory. Furthermore, his complex and sophisticated proposals are meant to deal with problems of efficiency and cost control that I believe are very real, very important, and not being dealt with now in the U.S. system. And lest anyone reply that these are someone else's problems, I further agree that the chances of getting more resources to improve the thoroughly unsatisfactory state of U.S. long-term care are remote indeed so long as U.S. government and private budgets are faced with the uncontrollable demands of the acute-care sector. The priorities may well be greater in long-term care, but no organization or group is likely to take on a second open-ended and uncontrollable commitment while the first is still an unsolved problem. Nor should they.

But in the spirit of advocacy, and in avoiding the academic problem of the "Uncertain Trumpet," AE may claim too much. (I believe he may also be a bit severe in his criticisms of publicly regulated systems like the NHS in the United Kingdom or the Canadian form of universal public health insurance.) In both cases, there are very real problems of innovation and of balancing citizen and provider interests, just as he points out, but the balance is not as one-sided as he suggests. Changes *have* been put through in Canada, like the recent suppression of extra billing, over the bitter opposition of physicians; and innovation *does* take place, albeit more slowly than in the United States. And one wants to be careful to compare the admittedly rather stodgy Canadian approach to change with the *realities* of the U.S. situation, not the idealized scenario that might emerge from "managed competition"—which is under examination in Canada as well. (We too read and listen to Alain!)

Feasibility

His proposals seem to me an excellent approach to health care funding—for people like himself. In his position, I would select the same option. And the competitive CMP with a responsible sponsor system may well be working for groups of people with the appropriate characteristics and as part of the community. What has not yet been shown is whether

1. the efficiency gains for individual groups generalize to the community as a whole
2. the sponsorship approach can be scaled up to universality without losing its essence

AE might (does) reply that a truly competitive system, in fact as opposed to rhetoric, has yet to be tried. I believe he is right. Present experience does not refute his approach—like Christianity (or Communism?), it has never been tried. But this leaves open two questions. Is it politically possible to make the changes necessary to give it a fair trial, and would it work then? I am at least uneasy on both counts.

But the status quo seems equally untenable. Though always the easiest choice for the short run, it may be the worst of all worlds in the long run. It may well be that, as suggested at the seminar, the proper course is for the United States to exploit its size, diversity, and federal structure and begin some experimentation at the state level. Perhaps California should be encouraged and assisted by the federal government to adopt AE's plan, while Massachusetts (say) adopts a version of a Canadian-style NHI program.

Some long-time supporters of federally based NHI, such as Rashi Fein, have now shifted, for several reasons, to advocacy of a state-based system. AE's insurer-of-last-resort role is located at the state level, and KD's expanded Medicaid system presumably remains state-based as well, although as I understand both of them, they would require considerably more standardization of benefits across states through increased federal regulation. Moreover, it may not be irrelevant that the Canadian system of health insurance is run at the provincial level, though supported by federal financial contributions and subject to some federal regulation of standards. Even more to the point, the pioneering plans were set up independently by certain provinces. When the federal legislation was passed, some years of working experience with universality at the provincial level was already in hand.

THE KANE PROPOSALS

This leads naturally into the consideration of Robert Kane's proposals, which are however much harder to critique. RK tends to enunciate general principles, which are on point, fundamental, and correct. But he does not go on to spell out detailed proposals, which makes the critic's job much more difficult. (Would that mine subject, certainly not enemy! had written a book. . . .) In particular, he stresses the fallacy of drawing sharp distinctions between public and private dollars and treating a public program as an extra expense to society if it merely transfers costs from private to public budgets (perhaps lowering them in the process). This logical and accounting fallacy does a great deal of harm in leading to erroneous evaluations; according to KD, however, it is simply part of the institutional reality and has to be accepted and worked with. How does one reconcile these two positions? RK is certainly right, but does that make KD wrong?

I suppose it emphasizes the educational task and possible contribution of a group such as AARP that could communicate the nature of this fallacy and, thus, improve the quality of public debate and decision making. It should not be too difficult for the members of AARP to see that a program that relieves them individually of some of the costs of long-term care and transfers these costs to government has not thereby added to the overall costs to American society, but has merely distributed them differently. Some may also object to that redistribution; but that is a different kind of issue.

RK also emphasizes the importance of rewarding quality of care based on outcomes, not merely the performance of procedures. All the other participants also stressed this point, though in KD's proposals it was difficult to see the institutional or behavioral link from improved insurance coverage to improved health outcomes. In fairness, the Canadian system suffers from exactly the same lack of linkage; access to care, as determined by professionals, is assumed equivalent to the promotion of health outcome, though we all know this is not true. AE goes further; his sponsors would have the responsibility for evaluating the effectiveness of care in terms of achieving outcomes and would have incentives to suppress ineffective care and promote only what is effective. The concern is that they would have other incentives as well, and it is not clear whether, in the end, they would promote efficient outcomes as diligently as claimed.

Interestingly, for RK, "the actual implementation of an outcome-monitoring system will require a special set of overseers, who will be a subset of those implementing the general program." Quite true, AE would call them sponsors. KD, more traditionally, would call them physicians. AE would, rightly, say that physicians do the job inadequately, for reasons not of personal inadequacy, but because of the structure and incentives within which they work. KD might reply that AE's sponsors would have similar problems; if so, I would agree. *Quis custodiet ipsos custodes?* RK does not provide a direct answer, but then neither did Plato. (Juvenal didn't think there was one.)

In Canada this responsibility is shared, insofar as it is taken up by anyone; the individual professional is responsible in the individual case, overseen by the hospital staff, if relevant, and the professional licensing bodies and the courts, but very loosely. The provincial government is ultimately responsible for the availability and scale of facilities and programs through its control of institutional budgets.

RK has some very positive things to say about the Canadian model, particularly the universality of public funding with private contracting to supply services by both not-for-profit agencies (hospitals) and for-profit ones (physicians and their practices). In particular, it corresponds to his comment about the maintenance of fee-for-service payment to providers, but not by consumers. In a very real sense, each Canadian provincial Ministry of Health is a geographically based HMO with a monopoly on the payment process (not the delivery system—we do not have socialized medicine). Each enrollee pays an amount through taxes and, in some provinces, premiums, that is related to his or her income, but not to either risk or experience of illness—an income-related, capitated payment. From this total sum, physicians are paid on a fee-for-service basis and hospitals on prenegotiated global budgets.

As AE says, there are no competitive incentives for efficiency, but that does not mean *no* incentives—just not many! Still, universality, cost control, and equity of funding distribution *are* achieved, without sacrifice of quality and effectiveness of care. (Canadian aggregate statistics on outcomes are slightly better than those in the United States and are improving at about the same rate.)

Kane's Long-Term Care

RK also makes some important general points about long-term care, particularly the dangers of "over-medicalization" and, yet, the need to rule out treatable organic problems in people in need of care. Some people may not need institutionalization or other long-term support if they can get better eyeglasses, or hearing aids, or simply take fewer drugs; and there is no substitute for a competent medical assessment. But beyond that, many of the problems of long-term care are not essentially medical; and it is a difficult trade-off as to whether long-term care is better provided through the medical system, where the resources are more extensive, or outside it, where they may be more appropriate. RK favors the model seen in some of the Canadian provinces, where long-term care is a public program with medical input, built on and presupposing a universal program of acute-care coverage but administered separately from the medical and hospital insurance programs.

In any case, RK says, and I agree, and so do AE and KD, the resources will have to be provided through public programs. Private long-term care insurance is simply a nonstarter for any significant share of the population. The only question is whether it is supported by taxes on the whole population or on the elderly subset. Can, and should, the elderly support such a program themselves, recognizing that whatever the eligibility for benefit (universal or age specific), it is almost exclusively elderly people who will benefit?

But which elderly? Predominantly those who are very elderly, over eighty-five. So why should the relatively arbitrary age of sixty-five be used as a definition of the tax base? I think there are good reasons for supporting the benefit out of general revenues—having it supported by the whole population—and this certainly is RK's view. But control of program costs will require, again, some form of overseer, or case manager, or sponsor, to determine who is eligible and for what, and to see to its purchase and provision. One is reminded of the United Kingdom's experiments with giving social workers budgets and requiring them to purchase care for their elderly clients.

The Overseer

The *Quis custodiet?* problem is universal in health care. RK suggests that with a proper structure for the case-manager role, which would reinforce changes currently taking place in the numbers and characteristics of the elderly, the nursing home industry as presently structured would virtually disappear. In its place could be a much more flexible and diversified system of alternative living arrangements supported by various forms of purchased services, either on call or periodic. RK does not, in this paper, provide the blueprint for such services but, rather, a set of principles that should govern their development. This is, of course, very far from his only work on the subject!

AGREEMENT IN DIVERSITY

Again, taking the papers together, (and implicitly including my own comments on the Canadian form of health care insurance and delivery), I am again struck by the extent of agreement in principle among an apparently diverse group of commentators. (AE in particular is sometimes described as rather right wing; he looks more like a center forward to me.) There was apparent unanimity on the desirability of universal and comprehensive coverage for acute medical and hospital care, with a distribution of the economic burden more or less according to ability to pay rather than on the spurious basis of "benefits received," spurious in this case because having to undergo treatment is *not* a benefit! There was, I think, equal though less explicit agreement on the need for some sort of agent to manage the access to and utilization of care by the individual, as well as the transactions in the insurance market. And there was certainly agreement in discussion, if not always explicit in print, that the *Quis custodiet* problem, of how to prevent abuse of this agency role, was present in all approaches in different ways.

The disagreements were over means, not ends, and had the following three sources

1. different hypotheses about the likely behavioral responses of the various participants—patients, providers, employers, and govern-

ments—in the health care funding and delivery process to changes in the institutional and incentive structure within which their interaction takes place
2. different degrees of emphasis on the seriousness of present or future shortcomings—the problem of inadequate access and unfair burden distribution, for example, as against that of waste, inefficiency, and ineffective servicing
3. different judgments about the political feasibility of alternative institutional changes, the strength and sources of resistance, the rigidities of the political process, and the possibilities of constituency building

From these differences emerged at least two radically different visions of the future of the U.S. health care system and two other less clearly articulated sets of principles and warnings. Yet, because they are each alternative means to similar ends, the proposals share a certain structural similarity in their responses to common questions. Their points of disagreement are genuinely open issues on which people of good will may reasonably differ and hope for resolution or, at least, clarification through discussion, debate, and evidence.

The time may be here, as well, for some large-scale experimentation—not in the formalized, randomized controlled-trial sense, which in the public policy arena often minimizes generalizability and global relevance even as it maximizes internal validity (a sort of Heisenberg principle in public policy?), but truly in the field, at the state level, exploiting the famous "social laboratory" possibilities of federal systems of government.

While "experimental," however, in the same sense that all human activity is so (we can always learn from experience, and sometimes even change), such state programs could not be partial or temporary but must be genuine policy initiatives. Saskatchewan was not "conducting an experiment," when they pioneered universal hospital insurance in 1946 or fought the medical profession, and won, to establish universal medical coverage in 1962. They were making decisions in real time, betting real careers, for real goals, with the intent that the world would be different and better thereafter. And it was.

Perhaps the last word in this commentary, then, should be Robert Kane's: ". . . A health care system must be based on a philosophic premise rather than on any set of research data. The latter are useful in examining alternatives and in guiding the implementation of a policy, but research will not lead directly to policy. . . . The transformation of the system will require a political act. It will follow a national expression of will."

AARP should participate in that expression.

INDEX